Praise for *It Sucked and Then I Cried*

"A frank and hilarious chronicle. . . . Her compassionate choice to share her experience will benefit many women and, more important, make them laugh."

—*Bust*

"Like her blog, [*It Sucked and Then I Cried*] is sometimes funny and irreverent, sometimes serious, and always honest."

—*USA Today*

"A funny, irreverent look at becoming a mother. The fact that it makes you laugh so often is quite a trick, since it is about, among other things, the postpartum breakdown that led to Armstrong's stay on a psychiatric ward a few months after [daughter] Leta was born."

—*The New York Times*

"Heather B. Armstrong is kinda like the Howard Stern of mommy bloggers."

—*Los Angeles Times*

"Feisty blogger and relapsed Mormon Armstrong takes her no-holds-barred approach to life from screen to page as she dishes on the elation, transformation, and despair that mark pregnancy, childbirth, and parenting. . . . A truthful picture of what it takes to bring a life into the world, exposing Achilles heels large and small."

—*Kirkus Reviews*

IT SUCKED

and then

I CRIED

How I Had a Baby, a Breakdown,
and a Much Needed Margarita

HEATHER B. ARMSTRONG

G

GALLERY BOOKS

New York London Toronto Sydney

For Mary Krause Fowler, the teacher who encouraged me to rhyme

G Gallery Books
A Division of Simon & Schuster, Inc.
1230 Avenue of the Americas
New York, NY 10020

First Gallery Books hardcover edition March 2010

GALLERY BOOKS and colophon are trademarks of Simon & Schuster, Inc.

For information about special discounts for bulk purchases,
please contact Simon & Schuster Special Sales at 1-866-506-1949
or business@simonandschuster.com.

The Simon & Schuster Speakers Bureau can bring authors
to your live event. For more information or to book an event
contact the Simon & Schuster Speakers Bureau at
1-866-248-3049 or visit our website at www.simonspeakers.com.

Manufactured in the United States of America

10 9 8 7 6 5 4 3 2 1

Library of Congress Cataloging-in-Publication Data

Armstrong, Heather B.
    It sucked and then I cried : how I had a baby, a breakdown, and a much needed margarita /
Heather B. Armstrong. — 1st Simon Spotlight Entertainment hardcover ed.
        p.   cm.
        1. Armstrong, Heather B.—Family.   2. Motherhood—Utah—Salt Lake City.
3. Salt Lake City (Utah)—Biography.   I. Title.
    CT275.A8219A3   2008
    306.874'3092—dc22
    [B]   2008038999
ISBN 978-1-4169-3601-5
ISBN 978-1-4391-7150-9 (pbk)
ISBN 978-1-4169-5914-4 (ebook)

Contents

Prologue

Many years ago I started a personal website so that I could share my thoughts on pop culture with a few of my friends scattered across the country. I wrote about movies and music and dissected the plot lines from short-lived sitcoms, sometimes adding a paragraph or two about the men in my life. Within a year my audience had grown from a few friends to thousands of strangers all over the world. More and more I found myself writing about my personal life, and eventually I started writing about my office job and how much I wanted to strangle my boss, often using words and phrases that would embarrass a sailor. When the company I worked for found my website, they fired me, walked me to my car with a cardboard box full of my belongings, and frisked me to make sure I hadn't stolen a stapler. Suddenly confronted with what I had done and who I had become, I took down my website because I knew I was about to have a nervous breakdown. And I didn't want to do it publicly.

Within six months I had put the website back online, although by that time I had learned to approach my writing with a heightened sensitivity to boundaries. I still wrote about my personal life, but I made sure to write about people in a way that they would never be upset when they showed up in one of my stories. Most of the stories at the time were about my new husband and how unemployment had forced us to move from Los Angeles to my mother's basement in Utah, and they would soon chronicle the purchase of our first house, the agonizing decision over paint chips, and the morning we saw a second line show up on a pregnancy test.

Pregnancy was an endless trove of content, and as my body changed I shared with my audience how I felt like I had been possessed by a hostile host organism. And although my website brought me a lot of comfort during those months, I truly believed that I would give it all up once I had the baby. I didn't think there would be time to maintain a website when my days would be filled with diapers and breast pads and hobbling to and from the crib.

But then I had that baby, and immediately everything in my life opened up with the same speed that it fell apart. My world expanded with a sympathy for every other human who had brought a child into their lives, but I had never before felt so isolated or alone. There were many days when the only way I could survive another hour was by writing about it.

So I kept writing about it, and then I had a nervous breakdown. Publicly.

The nine months of that pregnancy and the nine months after I brought the baby home were the most transforming period of my life. I had never flown so high, nor had I ever sunk so low. Hour by hour I searched for something to laugh about so that at the end of the day I could catch my breath instead of giving in to an overwhelming sense of hopelessness. A nuclear bomb had gone off in my living room, and although I had had nine months to prepare for the mess, it took me nine months to piece everything back together.

Luckily I collected notes throughout the cleanup, and when I finally stepped out of darkness and into daylight I realized just how close I had come to giving in, and how crucial it had been for me to share my journey. I don't think I would have survived it had I not offered up my story and reached out to bridge the loneliness. This is that story.

CHAPTER ONE

Let the Anxiety Commence

My husband has great hair, but even more impressive than that, he has impeccable taste in socks. And then there's his soft skin, pale white and scented with aftershave, always tempting me to press my nose in an ugly way to the side of his neck. He is a *good person,* someone who genuinely cares about other people and wants to see other people succeed. He loves his friends and his family, he doesn't cheat on his taxes, and he usually lets me have the last bite of ice cream. Most important, he has gigantic, bearlike hands, perfect for opening stubborn pickle jars and for holding me tightly when I'm freaking out.

His name is Jon, and together we had a baby.

I had wanted to be able to say that since our first date, a late breakfast at a dirty diner in Los Angeles a few years ago. I remember looking across the wobbly table, over a plate of bacon and buttered toast that I was too nervous to eat, and knowing that I wanted children with eyes like his, a piercing pale green. That afternoon after I said good-bye, after I kissed him gently next to the large swath of eyebrow that starts on one side of his head and continues uninterrupted across his forehead, I called my father and told him to write this name down: Jon Armstrong. Because he was the man I was going to marry.

A year later we eloped on a cliff at Yosemite National Park. It was a sudden decision, an idea we tossed around for barely a month, and we kept it secret from everyone we knew except his mother, and my mother, and my father. There was no way I could get married without telling my parents as I had put them through sufficient heartache already by leaving the Mormon faith that they had brought me up in, voting Democrat, and regularly reading Noam Chomsky. The best way I can describe the dynamic between me and my parents is that they would rather have me addicted to porn than donating money to the ACLU.

I remember calling my parents to let them know what we were doing, and I was a little nervous that my mother would freak out and try to talk me out of it, or maybe even hang up. But both of my parents were surprisingly thrilled that I was getting married. They thought it was the most responsible decision I had made as an adult, probably because it meant that they no longer had to be embarrassed that their youngest and wildest child was living in sin. Although, because I was not getting married in a Mormon temple, I was still throwing wrenches into their plans for me as a child, the biggest of which was that a non-temple wedding meant that I would not get to be with them in the hereafter and would instead end up in the part of Heaven reserved for thieves, murderers, rapists, and people who own autographed copies of Bill Clinton's head shot.

My parents have always loved Jon, sometimes more than they love me, and not just because it was mostly his idea for us to move to Utah to be closer to them. He is the more conservative one in our relationship, the one who is always turning down the radio, and I'm pretty sure that they think he saved me from living a long, lonely life by myself. Not because I don't have many great qualities, and I'll just go ahead and trot those out right now because my skill set is impressive. I have very nice elbows, not too pointy or too round. I can boil water. I can also parallel park a small car. Sometimes I am a nice enough person that I let someone else win at Scrabble. See?

My parents were worried that I'd end up a bitter spinster covered in cat hair because I inherited many of the annoying qualities of their own brothers and sisters. I can be loud and say inappropriate things, I will always laugh at a fart joke, and I often don't look in the mirror before I leave the house. But I am most like my aunts and uncles in that I have to take a lot of medication to prevent myself from throwing rocks at people. I suffer from chronic depression, and in the years before it was diagnosed I was a miserable human being who routinely wrote bad poetry about being misunderstood. I was a sophomore in college when it was finally treated, and I instantly became a much more bearable person, albeit one who had to pop a pill once a day to connect certain chemicals in my brain.

There are many people in my life who are embarrassed that I can freely admit this about myself, that I have to take pills to be happy, but before the pills I had tried a few of the other options that are out there for people like me:

1. I ignored that weird, sad feeling.
2. I substituted bad thoughts with thoughts of unicorns.
3. I exercised until the pain in my legs seemed far worse than the pain in my heart.

4. I overate to drown the sorrow.

5. I prayed that God would give me the will to get over it already.

Surprisingly, none of these things worked, and when I found myself on the brink of dropping out of college, my parents finally agreed to send me to a professional. After one week on an antidepressant I was a changed person, and I remained on that drug for the next seven years, right up until Jon and I got married. I stopped not because marriage had miraculously cured me of the grumples, but because I wanted to have a baby, had been jolted awake in the middle of the night for over a year by my biological clock screaming, "HEY! IT'S ME AGAIN! WHERE ARE THE BABIES?"

I wanted babies, so I stopped. At least, that's the medical term for what it's called, stopping. But I think they should call it Reenacting That One Scene From That One Movie Where That Guy Is Trying To Stop Using Heroin, and he's having a nightmare while he's awake that a dead baby is crawling across the ceiling, and he's all, oh God, oh God, please, please, make it stop, and the dead baby is twitching its rigor-morted head from side to side as it gets closer and closer, and then that guy throws up a hamburger.

Withdrawal from an antidepressant feels just like that, and in the first few months that I was off of my medication, I wanted to go back on almost every day. I needed the pills, because otherwise I did a lot of yelling and tossing things through the air, and sometimes Jon was an accidental target. Without my pills I was wildly irrational, and when we did not get pregnant THE FIRST MONTH WE STARTED TRY-ING, I was convinced that it meant I was barren. I saw the single line on the pregnancy test and fell into a giant wad on the floor because all I could imagine was years and years of fertility treatments that would never work, and if they did work it wouldn't be until I was sixty. And then we'd have quadruplets. And they'd all have fourteen toes. Because I wasn't good enough.

So we tried again the next month, and because I am a perfectionist driven to the point of madness with the need to be good at everything, I forced my husband to have a ridiculous amount of sex. One night after he had moved 7,800 pounds of boxes from a moving truck into our new house, I didn't even let him sit down to catch his breath before I had shoved him onto the bed and jumped on top of him like an alley cat might attack a discarded cheese sandwich.

"I'm ovulating," I told him as I tried to pry off his shirt.

"That's very sexy, and all," he said as he held his arms at impossible angles so that I couldn't get his clothes off. "But did you see what I just unloaded off that truck? IT WOULD TAKE AN ACT OF GOD, WOMAN."

But I didn't hear that. I heard: "You are ovulating, and I don't love you."

Because I am insane.

Two weeks later I took a second pregnancy test. I had promised myself that I was going to wait longer, just to give my body a little more time, but when Jon got up early one morning, I could only lie there alone for five minutes before giving in. I needed to know so that instead of having to experience all that torturous hoping, I could just go back to what I did best, being sad and worried about what it will be like to raise quadruplets in my sixties.

So I ran and got Jon, and we were like two ten-year-old kids digging through mom's closet to find Christmas presents. The second pink line on the test showed up within about four seconds, before I could even set it down on the countertop in the bathroom, and Jon and I nearly killed each other with hugs and screams and flailing, gangly arms. It was exactly like I had fantasized it would be in that I really did want to call every single person I knew, but the feeling itself was a single point of light swallowed almost whole by a vast space around it, like holy shit, we're going to have a baby! And at the same time, HOLY SHIT. WE'RE GOING TO HAVE A BABY.

Instead of getting into bed and going back to sleep after the 4 AM pregnancy test, we talked feverishly for three hours about what we were going to call our work in progress. It was a discussion I had waited my entire life to have, one that I had practiced hundreds of times before in my childhood with Barbies and Cabbage Patch Kids and a goldfish I accidentally boiled because I thought it would rather swim around in warm water. I know I'd much rather be warm than cold, why would my pet want anything different? Except once I put him in the water he started swimming in delirious circles, and then tried to JUMP OUT OF THE BOWL. TWICE. I sort of just stood there and watched him, like, fish is crazy! Until he turned upside-down and floated to the top. Maybe I won't repeat this story ever again, at least not until I have proven that *I know better now.*

I had hundreds of ideas for names, most of them stolen directly from the cast of *The Dukes of Hazzard* as there was no other show on television that has more accurately captured the spirit of my Southern upbringing, where my mama knew everyone's business and my cousins routinely took each other to prom. If my kid wasn't going to have my last name, he or she could at least look at their driver's license and be reminded of their maternal Tennessean heritage, one where wearing shoes to the grocery store is totally optional by law.

But giving a child the name Bo or Luke or even Rosco is way more generous to your offspring than naming your daughter after a character in a Western no one has ever seen whose most defining asset was that he shot a lot of people. That is what my father wanted to do, wanted to name my sister Mangus, even though that word sounds like a brand of cold sore. My mom didn't let this happen, but she did agree to let him name her September. Even though she was born in January. And my brother's name is Ranger. After a box of cigars my father saw at a truck stop in Arkansas. I guess this is one of the very few confounding things about my parents, that they are the most conservative people on the planet, and yet, the names of two of their children make them seem like Berkeley hippies who regularly dine on organic tofu.

Jon wanted nothing to do with a Bo or a Luke because he knew too many of those who had communicable diseases, and the act of calling our child one of those names would force him to lose four teeth. Which, okay, fine, we both had to agree on this, so I let him list his favorite names: SnigSnak, Qranqor, Styrofoam, KidNation, Frontline (after the television show or the flea medication), One (or First, or Premiere), Palette, Alphamask, Format (for a boy), Formatte (for a girl), Profile, Tweeter, Peavey. Possibly Wrench if the baby came out with an interesting nose.

While all of these ideas were teeming with originality and flair, two very important qualities in a baby name, we couldn't help but think that what our work in progress needed was something more Utahn. You cannot live in Utah and give your baby a boring name that some other baby in Wisconsin might have, and we couldn't get over the nagging feeling that someone in Wisconsin was naming their first-born child Alphamask as we lay there debating.

So in the tradition of the Utah Baby Name, we took an existing name and tweaked it into an unrecognizable mass of nonsense. It was not uncommon to meet people in this state who had names made up entirely of random letters just thrown onto either side of what could be, if you squinted hard enough, an actual word, like Aaronica or Ondulyn or Claravid. I threw out Fonzie which Jon transformed into Fawnzie, which when taken to its logical Utahn conclusion ended up being Fawnzelle. And so, our work in progress was called: Fawnzelle La Bon Marché Armstrong, if she turned out to be a girl; Fawnzel Le Bon Marché Armstrong, if he was a boy.

The middle name represented the European flavor we wanted to inject into the name, and even though I took four years of French in high school and two in college, the only French word I could think of other than croissant was Le Bon Marché, so it stuck. And I know that there is a good chance that I assigned the wrong gender to that word, but it didn't matter if it's a "le" or "la" because we were in Utah and no one would know the difference.

My family was horrified when I told them that I might actually do this to my child, and my sister, WHOSE NAME IS SEPTEMBER EVEN THOUGH SHE WAS BORN IN JANUARY, threatened to not talk to me again. This from a blond-haired, blue-eyed woman who named her two Aryan twins Noah and Joshua, after Jewish prophets. I am obviously the insane one in my family.

I thought I had prepared myself for the onset of nausea and fatigue and bloating and complete emotional instability of pregnancy by going through the agony that I did when I stopped taking an antidepressant, but during the first few weeks of pregnancy I could barely sit up straight without feeling the *thump thump thump* of my heart in my ears as it signaled the march of acid through my digestive tract, and it could not have possibly sucked more. It wasn't morning sickness, because the morning was over there in the front yard carrying on with its day while I was in the back of the house with my head in the toilet because some cosmetic company tried to jam every single smell of nature into one shampoo bottle, and then lie and call it an "essence." Those delicate little jasmine berries they add to make my hair smell like a fresh-cut flower reached out of the bottle while I was washing my hair and cut off my face with an axe.

Perhaps the worst smell I encountered during those first few weeks was the aroma of hand soap. I could not wash my hands without becoming hysterical, and the only reason we had any hand soap in the bathroom at all was because we needed to find a replacement soap, and that would involve walking into one of those bath and beauty stores, a veritable reservoir of insipid soap smells, a place where you can actually see the fragrance in the air, and for a pregnant woman that would be like walking into a gas chamber. Jon would often come back from the bathroom with hand soap stench on his hands, and it made me wonder whether or not he was intentionally trying to kill me. I know he was just practicing good personal hygiene, but it came down to a choice between his wife spontaneously gagging or having moderately dirty potty hands, and there I was, giving him permission to walk around with potty hands. Isn't that at the top of the list of what every man wants from his wife?

I blamed all those prehistoric women in caves who should have collectively decided that being nauseated like this *and* having to carry the baby at the same time is a raw deal. They should have put someone in charge of making some changes. And because they hadn't I decided I wasn't going to feel sorry for them anymore that sometimes they woke up in the middle of the night to find that a wild boar had eaten their cousin.

I cannot possibly forget what it felt like to be nauseated in my fingers and toes. The dizziness worked its way from the middle of my head down through every part of my body, and instead of feeling pregnant I just felt angry. I was mad that Jon could drink a beer and I was still able to smell it in his hair two days later. I was mad that a list of basic things that were a part of my daily life were forever going to remind me of the sensation of dry-heaving, like the smell of fabric softener, or the texture of chocolate pudding, or the way certain notes played over each other on the soundtrack to some of my favorite shows. Certain characters on some of my favorite shows would forever make me sick whenever I heard their voices, in particular a certain designer on a DIY home improvement show who glued things to walls that ought not have been glued to walls. Anyone idiotic enough to sign up for a reality television show probably deserves every injustice of life, but there are few sins in this world so evil enough that they warrant the punishment of having two tons of goose feathers hot-glue-gunned to the bedroom walls. And then there's that one episode where she wrapped a room in cardboard and made sure that even if the homeowners didn't want the walls of their guestroom covered in CARDBOARD, that there was no possible way they would ever be able to remove it because of all the nails and glue and tape and concrete she used to seal it to the drywall. That woman's face will from now on remind me of the inside of a toilet.

One thing no one ever told me about was that once I became pregnant I would experience a constant urge to go pee. I had no idea that during the early stages of pregnancy my bladder would spontaneously sprout its own holding tank, a reservoir of urine, so that God forbid I ever ran out of pee at any given moment I'd have at least a spare gallon standing by. Was that supposed to come in handy?

Going to the bathroom allowed me about thirty seconds of relief, a short half-minute of feeling like I didn't have to pee, and then once that minute ticked over into its second half my bladder would start billowing with the urge to go again. Given the era of technological innovation we live in, it wasn't terribly inconvenient for me to sit on the toilet all day long, as I had a laptop, a wireless Internet connection, and not one shred of dignity. However, venturing outside of the house was entirely problematic, as being any farther than an arm's length away from a bathroom triggered a battle of wills: my will vs. my bladder's will, and anyone who has ever challenged the will of an internal organ just trying to do its job knows that the internal organ always wins.

When I was at home I was peeing, and when I was away from home I was thinking about trying not to think about peeing. I *dreamt* about peeing. I even started asking pregnant strangers if they knew what I was talking about, which was dangerous for a couple of reasons. One: the only way I knew these women were pregnant was because they looked pregnant, and I was taking a huge risk in assuming that their giant bellies were filled with humans and not just a whole bunch of Oreos. Two: at some point my luck was bound to run out, and someone was going to knock me in the jaw when I walked up to them and asked them how often they used the toilet.

I picked up a few books and pamphlets here and there on the topic of pregnancy to see if I could find insight into this pee thing, because when coupled with the nausea, the inability to go more than ten minutes without a bathroom break was starting to give me second thoughts, like, *this is not at all what I signed up for!* and *what the hell have I done?* In my darkest moments, like the night I sprayed the backyard with staccato chunks of orange shrimp tikka masala, I wondered why women aren't equipped with tidy ctrl-z options, like, *undo eating that Indian food* or *undo biological urge to procreate.* There were countless mornings when I wished that I could have ctrl-z'ed the gel I put into my hair.

Nothing I had read up to that point in my pregnancy had done anything to make me feel better about the fact that I was facing months and months of ongoing discomfort. In fact, everything I'd read had the following wholly infuriating thesis statement:

Be careful and don't gain too much weight!

I am here to tell you that the last thing a pregnant woman in her first trimester wants to think about is how much weight she is gaining. Do you have any idea what *else* she has to worry about? According to the four books I had sitting on my nightstand, the list of things I had to worry about ran the gamut from not mixing certain household cleansers to not touching lunch meat with my bare hands else risking the possibility that the baby would be born with three ears. And if I touched a piece of sushi each of those three ears would be covered in scales.

What's even more annoying is that all those books began with a foreword in which the expert talked endlessly about how they planned to calm all the worries of an expectant mother, and then they spent the entire book detailing everything, real or imaginary, an expectant mother should be wary of. And every other sentence said something like, "Be careful and don't gain too much weight!" Always with the exclamation mark even though the word "weight" is already its own exclamation mark.

I will give them that it was hard not to think about the weight gain when I could feel my thighs separating at the joints. It was hard not to think about it when I could look at an entire chocolate cake and project manage in my head how I would get the entire thing down my throat in less than four minutes.

But on a good day I couldn't keep down a single meal without delivering it straight to the toilet wrapped in digestive acid, and I didn't understand why weight gain should be at the top of the list of things I was losing sleep over. AND I WAS TIRED OF READING ABOUT IT.

However.

My sister often brought over a pan of Rice Krispies Treats during those first few weeks, and although she told me she did this because she felt sorry for how sick I was, I know she did it to hurry along my massive weight gain. Because that's what siblings are for, to bring out the best in each other.

She knew that Rice Krispies Treats held the keys to my stomach. They are the world's perfect food: a mixture of cold cereal and butter, a transcendental blend of chewiness and crunchiness. In high school I used to make a whole pan of Rice Krispies Treats and then eat the entire thing by myself in less than a half hour. Of course, this was a time in my life when I was able to metabolize a cow by looking at it over a fence, and a 4,000-calorie pan of sticky breakfast cereal was just an appetizer before dinner.

I tried hiding them in dark corners of the basement, but I kept forgetting that I knew where I was hiding them, and I found them as soon as I hid them. I tried rationing them in little packages, but then I'd rationalize that each ration was lonely and needed friends, and so I'd eat four and five rations at a time. One time I gave up and just stood in the middle of the kitchen in my pajamas at four o'clock in the afternoon screaming at the pan, "STOP LOOKING AT ME!" Because their eyes were following me around the room.

The only other food I could even think about eating was a hot dog. In the seventh week of my pregnancy I ate more hot dogs than I had eaten in the collective whole of the rest of my life. I'm not talking about three or four hot dogs; I'm talking about the *whole package of hot dogs.* Hot dogs for snacks, hot dogs for lunch and dinner, hot dogs on the way back from each of the four pee breaks in the middle of the night.

Also, sauerkraut. For breakfast. Because the box of salt I ate before-hand wasn't salty enough.

At the beginning of my eighth week of pregnancy I experienced a rare morning when I was able to walk around and perform normal tasks without wanting to puke my spleen through my nose. I was smiling, and there was a noticeable lilt in my step, and it all felt completely un-natural. I'd forgotten what it was like to be okay, and I was so happy to feel okay that I even thought about washing my hair. I was almost out of control.

I felt so good that I thought I'd spend some time with our dog, Chuck, a one-year-old brown mutt that we had adopted from a shelter in Los Angeles. He resembled almost every dog imaginable, and you could see Jack Russell terrier in his face, pit bull in the shape of his body, yellow Labrador in his ears, and greyhound in the speed with which he could outrun other dogs. His favorite activity was meet-ing other dogs, so I put him in the car and drove to the dog park, which totally astounded him because he'd become used to seeing me lying under a bundle of covers in the dark bedroom, twitching and moaning and mumbling some nonsense about how much it sucked to be a woman. Chuck often looked at me, in between bites of a stuffed toy, like he understood, like he was sorry I had to suffer painful bloating and sore boobs—so sore that the resulting breeze from shutting the refrigerator door made me feel like a baby seal being clubbed by poachers.

Chuck chased a chocolate Labrador from one end of the park to the other, and after we walked back to the car I coaxed him into drinking a small handful of water to cool off from all the activity. Once we climbed back into the car we both hung our heads out of the window to feel the wind in our faces, and you couldn't have found two happier companions, happy to be alive and feeling okay. I was feeling so okay that I ignored the splash of water I suddenly felt scatter across my face and upper body, blaming it on a sprinkler we might have passed or maybe a small rain shower. And I was still feeling happy and okay when I noticed out of the corner of my eye that the dog was chewing on something, and I thought, isn't that nice? The dog is *so cute* when he chews on something.

I finally turned my head to notice that the dog was chewing malformed bits of apples and peanut butter THAT I HAD FED HIM THAT MORNING, and my brain was so rattled from the pregnancy that it took several seconds for me to put together what had happened, that while his head was hanging out the window, the small handful of water got together with the apples and peanut butter and planned an explosive revolt out his snout. And the water and the apples and the peanut butter hit the air whooshing past the window and splattered all over the inside of the car, all over the outside of the car, all over his face and all over my right arm. And he was just sitting there chewing regurgitated bits of apple and peanut butter as they dripped off his ears and chin. As if that's what you're supposed to do when you throw up your breakfast into your own lap.

Owning a dog is nothing like raising a child, but I can confidently say that I felt exactly like a parent when I pulled the car over in the middle of downtown Salt Lake City and picked *someone else's* puke out of every crack and crevice of that car. And yet, that type of chaotic situation was not an anomaly with Chuck, and since the day that we adopted him from the SPCA in Pasadena, California, I had rarely *not* felt like a parent.

During the first six weeks of Chuck's life we were unsure whether or not we'd actually adopted a dog and not some sort of abandoned scientific experiment, perhaps a hyena crossed with a mountain lion crossed with a mythical Latin goat sucker. He was four weeks old when we brought him home, and so all those little life lessons he should have learned from his brothers and sisters during the first eight weeks of his life, like not biting, and understanding that when someone else yelps they're saying, *stop it, you're hurting me*, all those little nasty feral dog habits were left up to us to cure. And because the experience of bringing him home was such a shock, one that I never wanted to live through again, a certain part of me feared that when we brought home our baby it would immediately start to crawl around and bite our ankles.

I had never had a dog before Chuck, wasn't allowed to own anything other than a fish—which I boiled accidentally, have I mentioned that?—because, according to my father, animals do not poop little poop, and as far as my father is concerned there is no such thing as a bodily function. "Because they don't poop little poop" would become the answer to every request I made for most of my childhood. I couldn't stay out past midnight because my boyfriend didn't poop little poop. Couldn't go to Florida on spring break because people in Florida didn't poop little poop. The plot of that rated R movie I wasn't allowed to see? It was all about big poop.

And since Chuck was the first animal I had ever owned, I had no idea what to do with him, starting with how to get him to stop biting me, something that was happening almost every second he was awake, on the fingers, on the ankles, on the elbows. He even managed to bite me on the forehead once, as I was leaning down to tell him to stop chewing on my underwear.

I read tons of books and websites, some of them written by pacifist monks, some of them written by sergeants in the U.S. military, to try to learn how to be a good dog owner. All of them claimed that their method was the best method, and that if I didn't follow their method then I might as well just give up now because my dog would inevitably bite the fingers off starving, innocent children. I find that instructional literature about parenthood is almost exactly the same in that every expert thinks all the other experts are out of their minds. How could they possibly come to *that* conclusion when the book you have in your hands is based on an entirely different and contradictory conclusion? No one agrees on anything except that everyone else is deranged, and I get the feeling that not one of these experts has been laid since graduate school.

The general consensus among dog-training experts, however, is that no matter what method dog owners choose, they have to prove to the dog that they are the alpha dog in the pack, the leader, the one who calls

all the shots. And in those very early months I tried telling that to
Chuck. I tried to alert him in an authoritative voice that I was the big
dog in this relationship. And you could tell, if not from the bearing of
his fangs then from the gaping scar he left on my shin, that he took me
very seriously.

So we tried more physical methods of demonstrating our alpha-ness,
like flipping him over on his back and gripping his jowls like his mother
might do. We tried barking and baring our teeth. I even tried *biting him
back.* But nothing worked until we spent a large sum of money on a
trainer who came into our house and used a few small gestures, including a convincing impression of Darth Vader, to let Chuck know that he
was the dog and that everyone else was human. That trainer taught me
how to walk the dog, how to get him to sit, to stay, to come, and I remember the first time Chuck ever took a long nap, about a month into
his training regimen. It was during the late-morning hours when he was
usually sprinting laps around the kitchen or swiping the remote control
to gnaw on it underneath the bed. Finding him prostrate, I thought
something was wrong with him, thought maybe he was sick or dying,
because he had never before sat still, had never willingly remained in a
horizontal position. I called the trainer crying, like, *oh my God, I should
never have adopted this dog because I have no idea what I'm doing and now
he's dead and I killed him.* And the trainer, who I now realize was my life
coach, just laughed and said, "Dogs sleep. That is what they do." And
I was all, if this is what dogs do, then I'll take ten, please.

That first morning nap that the dog took was a turning point in my
relationship with Jon, because I felt like I finally had a grip on taking
care of another creature, that I could finally let myself feel the fullness
of wanting children. I really believed I could do it, because the joy of

having the dog around had become bigger than the pain of it, and there was a lot of pain. There were two months of housebreaking, of running fifty feet along a hallway, down a flight of stairs, and then across a parking lot to a tiny patch of grass EVERY HOUR FOR SIXTY STRAIGHT DAYS. I remember thinking that there was no way potty-training a toddler could be worse than that, and that I'd personally invest money in the company that invented diapers for dogs, just so that I could sleep through the night.

There was that one time when Jon spilled a bag of coffee beans and thought he had cleaned up the mess, but he hadn't cleaned up the mess at all whatsoever, and Chuck hunted out and swallowed every last stray coffee bean, and the consequent twelve hours were The Worst Twelve Hours of My Life, ending only when his buzz ended.

Or the time he became infected with the world's worst case of fleas. I happen to know that it was the world's worst case because any case of fleas involves actual fleas, and even if only one flea were involved it still would have been a flea, and therefore, the worst possible scenario in the universe. It was a few months before we left California, and had we been living in Utah this never would have happened as fleas cannot live at such an elevation. The only thing a dog can really catch outdoors in Utah is heartworm and a healthy testimony of Jesus Christ.

One afternoon while the dog and I were playing tug of war on the living room floor, I noticed that his fur was moving. At first I thought that I had brushed his fur in the wrong direction, and there it was working its way back into place. But then it would move back into the wrong position, and the effect made his body look like it was trying to say something to me. Like, DEAR HUMAN, THIS IS NOT RIGHT.

When I closely inspected the fur behind his ears I distinctly saw a flea staring me squarely in the eyes, and the first thing that came to my mind was:

Let's try to vacuum the fleas off of his body.

Seemed reasonable. They'd pop off his fur. Just like that. Why had no one thought of this before me?

It would be easy. One of us would hold Chuck down while the other took the vacuum hose and suctioned off the fleas. Since I was the one who was at home with the dog most of the day, I decided that I would be the one to hold him down, reasoning that my embrace would be comforting and familiar. But I forgot that I was hyperventilating and on the verge of a panic attack. There were fleas in my apartment near my underwear. I would have been more comfortable having my front teeth tied to the back of a moving pickup.

Once I had Chuck in a cradled position, my arms trembling with the thought of what was crawling around so close by, Jon turned on the vacuum cleaner and slowly approached us. And to me it just sounded like a vacuum cleaner; to Chuck it sounded like, "Oh my God, it's The End of the World and it is SCREAMING AT ME." Jon was only able to suction a tiny square inch of fur on Chuck's stomach before Chuck turned into an African cheetah and clawed out of my arms. He immediately ran yelping into the bathroom carrying his flea-infested ass to the place where my body got naked to take showers.

Hours later, after the fleas had multiplied and established a thriving metropolis in Chuck's nether regions, we stuck him in the bathtub and atom-bombed their command center. When the tub drained there were literally thousands and thousands of dead fleas clinging to the porcelain, and it was my job to clean up the mess. I did it dutifully like any parent would, and like my own parents used to torture me, I would occasionally taunt Chuck mercilessly by breaking out the vacuum cleaner and leaving it sitting upright next to his head while he slept.

Having Chuck in our lives made us feel a little wiser, a little more understanding of what every other dog owner was living through. And in many ways I understood that having a child would increase our sympathy for other people in exactly the same way, and that in no time we'd be walking around comparing the war wounds on our shins and heels with everyone else who had made it out alive.

CHAPTER TWO

How to Exploit an Unborn Baby

When Jon and I got back from my twelve-week checkup where we heard the baby's heartbeat for the first time, it was hard to comprehend what I was feeling, a mixture of disbelief and fear, excitement, a little bit of heartburn, definitely some nausea, but I knew undoubtedly that those little thumping pulses would make it possible for me to go another day hunched over the toilet with half of my internal organs lodged in my esophagus.

It had been four weeks since I'd first seen my doctor, and I'd gained back four of the ten pounds I lost in those first few weeks of pregnancy. My guess was that those four pounds were made up entirely of hot dogs, refried beans, sauerkraut, and Nacho Cheese Doritos. Sadly, everything you've ever heard about pregnant women and cravings and the complete erosion of decency is absolutely true, and one embarrassing Saturday night I found myself standing utterly defenseless in line at Kentucky Fried Chicken ordering Extra Crispy chicken wings and buttermilk biscuits. Honestly, that was the only thing I could have eaten at that moment, fried chicken made specifically by the Colonel, and I couldn't remember a better tasting meal in the last ten years of my life.

Another change since that first visit to the doctor was all my clothes started to fit *differently,* even though I was still five pounds under my normal weight. I couldn't wear any of my jeans anymore, and even the baggy pants in my wardrobe were too tight to zip up. I still refused to buy any maternity clothes, however, because I was morally opposed to wearing any sort of clothing that by design invited strangers to coo and put their hands on my belly. There would be no cooing in my presence, and for crying out loud, NO BELLY TOUCHING.

I definitely thought that the nausea would have begun to subside by week twelve, but that week was by far the worst of the whole pregnancy up to that point. And there is no way to describe what that type of nausea felt like, just how tortured I was by that sickness. And whenever people would ask me, always expecting me to nod quickly in return, "Don't you love being pregnant?" I felt like I needed to stand up for every woman who has thought to herself in dark moments that being pregnant is the worst lot in life and give them a lengthy, gory, detail-ridden treatise on why in reality the whole process mostly sucked, starting with what it tasted like to puke up banana pudding.

The nausea had also caused me to loathe the smell of alcohol, and when Jon drank beer he was not allowed to sleep in the house. When Jon first moved in with me, about two and a half years before I got pregnant, we began consuming alcohol and coffee in very large quantities. I don't think either of us had been very big alcohol or coffee drinkers up until that point, but there was something about the giddiness we felt when we were around each other that brought out the naughty juvenile in both of us. We had in common a rather stringent Mormon

upbringing that forbade us the enjoyment of alcohol or any hot, caf-
feinated beverage, and I think we went about drinking both together
like bandits, relishing with flagrant naïveté the sinful buzz brought on
by liquids that will drown the soul to Hell.

I'd be terrified to see an X-ray of my liver because when I say that we
began drinking on a very daily basis, I mean *very* daily, more daily that
just your normal, average daily. We drank alcohol every day, multiple
times during the day, multiple drinks multiple times during the day.
And we never consumed beer or cider or anything that would require
more than one refill in order to get a stinking buzz. We drank bourbon
on the rocks, or straight shots of tequila, or double vodka martinis. We
drank on empty stomachs, before sundown, often after vigorous workouts, before rehydrating with water. I'm quite certain that during those
workouts anyone standing next to us could smell the bourbon in our
sweat.

Drinking as much as we drank wasn't necessarily the smartest or
healthiest way of living, although it did make watching the first install-
ment of *American Idol* a deeply spiritual, highly interactive experience.
It also made for extraordinary hangovers—aching, screaming, gut-
eating hangovers—that lasted weeks, even months at a time. All of that
stopped when we found out I was pregnant, and Jon showed his soli-
darity by joining me in abstinence, or at least frequent abstinence punc-
tuated by the occasional Bud Light. And on those occasions I could
smell the beer in his pores, and then I'd have to dry heave for several
hours. Alcohol was surprisingly one of the easiest habits I'd ever had to
give up, much easier than kicking a nasty Diet Dr Pepper addiction I
had my freshman year in college when I would refill a sixty-four-ounce
mug three to four times a day just to stay awake through Calculus.

In those two or three seconds where we heard the trumpeting

cadence of life growing in my abdomen, I completely believed all the hype, that the whole mess, the never-ending nausea, the tightening of my favorite jeans around my expanding hips, the craving of all things Kentucky Fried, the grinning and bearing it when Jon couldn't resist happy hour, it was worth it. We were going to have a baby.

Although I didn't think I would ever feel better, I woke up at the beginning of my fourteenth week of pregnancy feeling remarkably fine. I really did believe that I was going to be sick the entire pregnancy, and then afterward for the rest of my life because I'm optimistic like that. I come from a long line of Southern women who were sick the entire nine months of their pregnancies, my mother and sister included, and although I was the first woman in my family stubborn enough to reject the whole notion of panty hose, I suspected that I would be forced through defective genes to suffer forty weeks of incessant gut-churning, face-contorting, Nacho Cheese Dorito-laden vomit.

My nausea only lasted thirteen weeks, exactly as long as my doctor said it would. But I hadn't been able to take my doctor seriously, primarily because he introduced himself to Jon by saying, "Last time she was in here she didn't know who the father was. Have you guys figured that out yet?"

That type of bedside manner may be funny on a sitcom where a famous actress is pregnant *with a pillow stuck up her shirt,* but in real life, the kind of real life that involves me and my superparanoid husband of fiery Scottish descent who is about to hear his child's heartbeat for the very first time, this type of bedside manner CAN CAUSE A HEART ATTACK.

This is the same doctor who told me that the only thing he could prescribe for nausea was an anal suppository—you know, the type of suppository that has to be inserted anally, *that* type of anal suppository. Maybe I should take a sentence or two here to summarize why I am not fond of anything that might exacerbate my lifelong battle with constipation and how, from time to time, more often than not, especially during the first months of pregnancy as the entire chemistry of my body morphed spasmodically into a host organism, I lost all ability to poop.

Sometimes I just misplace the ability like I misplace car keys, under the bed or in between the cushions in the sofa, and after a few hours of looking I'm back to normal and can start the car again. But usually my ability to poop goes missing entirely, not unlike Jimmy Hoffa, disappearing without a trace, perhaps to pursue a life in hiding, more likely than not abducted and killed by the Mafia.

I am the only one of my mother's three children who was breastfed, and she says it's because I was born at a time when it was in vogue for women to formula feed their children. Since I am the youngest and last child, she decided that she wanted to try breastfeeding with me. Almost two years after I was born she still couldn't decide if she would ever stop, and the result? Her only breastfed child grew up to be a wayward Democrat, whereas the other two are God-fearing, law-abiding Republicans. I can see the correlation clearly.

I'm also the only one who has suffered chronic constipation her entire life, and although I'm no doctor and rarely have any idea what I'm talking about, I like to think that it goes all the way back to the first couple weeks of my life. I didn't have a normal bowel movement for fourteen days after I was born, and even though my mother called the pediatrician several times, concerned that something was wrong with my inner workings, he assured her that this was normal and that I would grow up a healthy, intact kid with normal plumbing, albeit one who would eventually grow up and vote for Ralph Nader.

As it turns out, I'm a pretty healthy kid, moderately intact and surprisingly good with multiplication tables. But there is nothing normal about my plumbing. Those first fourteen poopless days did something awful to my body, and I have suffered constipation nearly constantly since then. I remember my fifth birthday party when I swallowed over two hundred gumballs in less than a half hour, a strategy I employed to keep my older brother from stealing any of them. Seven days later my mother sat on the edge of the bathtub holding both of my hands, coaching me through pain management techniques as each gumball tried to find an exit out of my body. I think I pushed so hard that they eventually came out of my foot.

During the first year that I lived in Los Angeles I reintroduced meat into my diet after eight years of being a strict vegetarian *while I had guests staying with me for the weekend.* Which I guess is like saying, sure, come stay with me, but I won't be able to hear a word you're saying over the sound of my body yelling at me.

After a particularly filling meal of steak and potatoes on the third evening of their stay, I spent over two hours in the bathroom praying that God might spare my life and let me return to the guests waiting in the living room. I finally had to call my boyfriend, have him drive across town to my apartment, and then barricade him in the bathroom where I whispered, "You're going to have to get me an enema because otherwise I won't come out alive." Is it really possible to whisper *enema*? Doesn't that word demand to be cried maniacally through gnashing teeth?

My boyfriend then walked several blocks down to a drugstore in the most homosexual neighborhood in Southern California and bought two Fleet Enemas "for my girlfriend back home." I only like telling this story because the cashier at the drugstore gave him a subtle indication that he did not believe him, and this rankled my boyfriend so badly that he remained there at the checkout arguing with the cashier so long—"No, really, she's my *girl*friend!"—that by the time he got back to my apartment, my guests had gone to bed. AND I WAS STILL IN THE BATHROOM.

My system is so sensitive that if my daily routine varies even slightly my body forgets how to poop. I have to drink two cups of coffee at the same time every morning, have to consume at least a half gallon of water and eat at least one bowl of bran-infused cereal a day. At four o'clock every afternoon I stand in the middle of the backyard, hold my arms out perpendicular to my body, turn three circles to the left, then one to the right, touch my toes and clap my hands twice. If I forget and only clap my hands once I don't poop. If the wind changes direction I don't poop.

And when I was pregnant, none of those rituals mattered. In fact, I would not have been surprised if the pregnancy had made it so that I wouldn't ever poop again, and if that was the case, what do you know! Something else no one was willing to warn me about.

Once I started to feel better Jon and I made a point of leaving the house more often. One night very early in my second trimester we attended a concert by musician Norah Jones at a venue in an open field on the side of a mountain overlooking the Salt Lake Valley. Seating at this venue was general admission, meaning normally we would sit wherever we could find a patch of grass, but that night we got to sit in the VIP section, a small rectangular area directly in front of the stage with upright white folding chairs, because our friend knew the drummer in Norah's band. That did not stop me from telling everyone around us that it was because I was pregnant, and I was horrified when those words came out of my mouth. I couldn't stop them, it was an urge I could not stifle, something inside that made me want those people to understand that being pregnant made me special. And after I said it I remembered why I find pregnant women so annoying.

It was the first real outing we'd taken since the beginning of the pregnancy, and for two exquisite hours we sat facing the middle of the stage while sucking watermelon Jolly Ranchers, a suitable alternative to white wine, and listened to Norah's voice drip like honey onto sandpaper. It was one of those sublime Utah summer nights where it's almost chilly enough for a sweater, but warm enough that you can smell the neck of the lover sitting beside you, and the sun fell behind the mountains to the west in electric bands of neon color.

The venue was packed with earthy non-Mormon Utah types, people who live here despite, not because of, the religion. Everyone had some sort of alcoholic beverage in their hand, something they'd brought from home or bummed off the person sitting next to them, mostly white or red wine, a pint of lager here and there. And that was precisely why it had been so hard for us to go out those first few months of my pregnancy, because the smell of people partying was right up there with sewage.

The VIP section of the crowd was a virtual who's who of Utah celebrity. Although I was disappointed that there was no Osmond sighting, we sat directly behind a local news anchor who had one of the most beguiling mustaches on the planet, and in a state where facial hair was considered an outward signifier of "evildoing," those of us who did evil on a regular basis appreciated his high-profile representation. Plus, he wasn't wearing socks, so we could see his ankles. And because he was showing so much skin I could totally imagine what he would look like naked.

The concert itself was phenomenal, full of every hit song she'd ever written plus a few covers of some country classics, and Norah's voice was a thousand times more remarkable than any live recording could ever capture. After she played her final song we followed our friend to the after-show party at a large greenhouse up the hill from the venue. The room was littered with half-eaten food, and within seconds of stepping foot in the building the pregnant demon inside of me couldn't keep its face out of the cheesecake. There I stood surrounded by members of Norah's band, civilized people who use words like "amenable" and talk about NPR, and instead of making small talk or doing my best impression of an evolved person, I stuffed my face with stale cheesecake, skipping utensils and napkins altogether. I also stole a forty-dollar bottle of chardonnay out of their cooler, something I planned to drink a year and a half later when I'd weaned the baby off breastfeeding, or perhaps sooner if I mastered the whole horrific pumping mechanism. All I knew is that I would one day be able to drink alcoholic beverages again, and when that day came, what better way to celebrate than with an illicit bottle of wine I'd poached from a rock star with great tits?

The wait staff eventually had to tear the cheesecake platter out of my trembling hands to clean up for the evening, so I jumped into a conversation my husband was having with Norah's drummer and guitarist, two very lovely, sickeningly talented people who were way too sober to be on tour. So lovely and talented were they, in fact, that when the gui-

tarist reached out and touched my belly, WITHOUT MY PERMIS-
SION, twice within the span of five minutes, neither Jon nor I bit his
hand off or broke his arm.

After about an hour of milling about the after party and talking with
the band, wherein Norah appeared and disappeared three or four times,
everyone headed outside to wait for the VIP golf cart to show up and
take everyone back to the tour bus. The drummer suggested that we
wait with the band instead of walking all the way back to the parking
lot, but Jon, not wanting to appear a mooch, refused the offer, saying
that we'd be fine walking back by ourselves. I, however, considered
mooching to be an art form and instantly mentioned to the drummer
that I was pregnant and probably shouldn't walk back in the dark because that would be bad for the baby. I figured, I'm only going to be
pregnant two or three or seven times, and if my baby is going to use me
for nutrients for the next five months, why not use it to score a golf-cart
ride with Norah Jones? I can guarantee you that any child of mine
would see the logic in this reasoning.

So the golf cart showed up, and everyone in the band piled on, except for the drummer who gave up his seat so that I didn't have to walk.
And it turned out there wasn't enough room for Jon anyway, so he got
to walk back in the dark, content in not having had to mooch, man-
hood still intact. But I climbed up on that golf cart and sat directly
behind Norah, who looked back at me and smiled like, "I'm smiling
because I'm friendly, not because I have any idea who you are."

She then asked, "Are you the one who's pregnant?"

And I knew that she could see straight through me, could see that I
was a mooch and that I was so much of a mooch that I would use my
unborn baby to score a ride on a golf cart with her, and I nodded, afraid

that if I opened my mouth to say anything, the blood I'd been sucking from her band members all night might drip from my vampire fangs.

So she turned back around, and the golf cart started motoring down the mountain, as fast as its little golf cart motor could go. And the moon was bright, and the breeze was perfect as it moved down the canyon, and I was sitting behind Norah Jones on a golf cart. All I could think about was how, maybe twenty years from that moment, I would have at least one story to tell my child that would make me, if only for a very brief moment, the cool one.

Thirty seconds into the ride as we rounded a tree-covered corner, about seven members of the tour group—roadies and managers and sound technicians—all came screaming out of the bushes like crazed, ferocious werewolves in an attempt to scare the life out of Norah. Consequently, the golf cart almost careened off into a ravine, and that bowel movement I hadn't had in two years seemed like it might enter stage left.

After everyone on the golf cart regained composure, Norah turned around, eyes on FIRE, the hair on the back of her neck standing straight on end, and she reached back to cover my stomach and screamed, "THIS WOMAN IS PREGNANT, YOU IDIOTS!" Like she was my protector, my angel sent from heaven.

I felt so accepted in that moment, so understood. She was the rock star, and I was the lowly mooch who had pilfered a bottle of wine from her stash. Yet, she overlooked all of that because of my pregnancy, because of my tiny round belly. And when I met back up with Jon at the bottom of the hill I told him everything, including the part about how I had gone flying through the air, and how Norah had caught me in her arms before I landed in a giant pit of alligators.

CHAPTER THREE

A Twenty-pound Basketball
With Legs and Arms

When I was four months pregnant I walked up to a mirror, turned to the side, and stared intently at my belly to inspect the growth. Maybe it's because I'm five feet eleven inches tall, and every feature of my body is elongated, but instead of looking pregnant, I only looked painfully bloated.

But my boobs? Wow. My boobs were the most glaring side effect of second trimester pregnancy. I thought maybe I was the only one who noticed until we had dinner with my sister one night, and the first thing she said to me, very loudly, in front of all of her children and six of my visiting aunts and uncles, was, "My little sister grew boobs!" As surprised as if the same change had happened to our brother.

She had every right to be alarmed by the new set of appendages sitting on my chest. My small-chestedness had been a stabilizing constant in our family's lives, not unlike their belief that the Mormon Church was true and that God lived. They had always been able to testify with very much faith and confirmation from the Spirit that Heather had no boobs, in the name of Jesus Christ, Amen.

I marveled at my new boobs daily, primarily because I'd always wanted boobs, more than I ever wanted Malibu Barbie or front row tickets to a Debbie Gibson concert. If the eleven-year-old Heather had known that the much older, pregnant Heather was going to have such cleavage, she never would have worn that poorly designed padded bra for so many months, and the endless teasing and torment, which included being pelted with tissue paper every time I got on or off the bus to middle school, never would have happened. If I had only known that my profile in my second trimester of pregnancy would include bumps other than my nose and chin, I could have saved thousands on psychotherapy.

Another less satisfying side effect of having made it through those first three months of nausea was that I was able to eat properly for two, and once I was done with two I fed the other fifteen appetites that had seemingly taken over my personality. There are no words to describe the hunger I experienced at any given moment, and not even white bread could satiate the urge to eat my own fingers. Not that I didn't try to curb the demons with white bread—croissants, crumbly buttermilk biscuits, hot buttered rolls, English muffins, an entire loaf of Wonder Bread. I felt only a little guilty for clogging my arteries with enough carbohydrate voltage to power the western United States, and I became convinced that if the battery on our car were to die we could have jump-started it by hooking a set of cables up to my chest.

In addition to my new boobs and the crippling hunger, the major second trimester side effects I experienced were the aches and pains and cramps associated with the expansion of my uterus. I slept on my left side the entire night and could physically feel my thighs stretching and cracking in opposite directions. My hips moved so significantly that the only thing I could wear was sweatpants, but because I refused to buy maternity sweatpants they were always slipping off my butt. I dealt with this by holding up my pants with one hand while using the other hand to pull my shirt down over my bare belly, and I'd walk around hunched over like a paranoid lunatic who had eaten too many cupcakes at lunch.

And it's not that I was necessarily opposed to showing off my pregnant belly in public, but I learned quickly that the practice of belly exposure only enticed strange people to walk up and put their hands on my body. Unfortunately, strange people make up about 90 percent of the population in Utah, and they all stared at my bare belly like it was some sort of sacred Budha that would release the secrets of the world if they just walked up and rubbed it. The only thing going on behind the cherubic curve of my belly was the sound of a digestive tract processing four thousand Nacho Cheese Doritos that I'd eaten after lunch.

I kept hearing that the second trimester was the best trimester because, hey look! No more morning sickness! Also, you're not yet as big as a Hummer! But did you know this? The second trimester is basically puberty ALL OVER AGAIN, as if the first time wasn't painful enough. My body felt totally awkward, as if I'd just grown four inches in eighteen months again, except this time the four inches were at my waistline, and pants that fit fifteen minutes ago were suddenly cutting off oxygen to the baby.

I didn't "get out of" bed anymore, either. Getting out of bed was more of an assisted roll and shove off the mattress where Jon pushed my backside with his arms and legs using a strength he'd normally reserved for knocking over a brick wall. And the acne! Those were not your aver-age, friendly variety of pimple. They were pregnant pimples, deposits of hormonal oil embedded so deep in the skin that I didn't know whether I had a tick rooting through my forehead or an alien pod trying to free itself out the middle of my back.

I felt really sorry for Jon, because I knew he fully expected my head to start spinning all the way around and for his dead ancestors to start speaking through my mouth. All he could do was watch this terrifying metamorphosis take place from a safe distance, preferably behind a stain-resistant protective wall. The good news was that we were almost halfway through the whole mess, only twenty or so more weeks to go. The bad news was that he had to spend those twenty weeks *married to me.*

Five months into the pregnancy we found out whether we were having a boy or a girl, or God forbid one of each or two of one. I think my fears of giving birth to multiple babies may have been a little more profound than the average pregnant woman, as twins run rampant in both Jon's family and in my own: my sister has twin boys, Jon's sister has twin boys, two of my cousins have sets of twins, and one cousin has two sets of twins. My family thought it would be awfully cute if I, too, had twins, and I just thought it would be awfully awful.

During the first trimester I was convinced that I was having a boy, primarily because I only had dreams about boys and I also craved spicy food. Most of the men in my life love to torture themselves by dousing their dinners in hot sauce or by eating jalapeño peppers whole, without water or fire extinguisher. It could be one of the reasons I fell in love with my husband, that he is so much like my father when he looks for the one item on the menu that is most likely to burn a hole in the side of his mouth. They both get giddy with the possibility of a meal rendering them unconscious, as if the more sweat they bleed from their forehead during a meal, the more they can provide for their families.

I'd never understood this ritual, as I like to eat my meals in relative comfort, without fear of imminent death, until I got pregnant. Once I had a baby to think about it was as if I needed to prove to the baby, to myself, and certainly to the wait staff that I could withstand the burning flames of spicy food, if only to demonstrate that I was going be a good mother. The two have nothing to do with each other, I know this, but I guarantee that many men will totally understand this line of reasoning.

We did not care about the gender of the baby going into the ultrasound, and I know that everybody says that, or is at least *supposed* to say that. But since this was our first we had no practical experience to tell us what would make one preferable over the other. Although, I did contemplate what a delight it would be to horrify my feminist, graduate student friends by imposing my stringent, close-minded, puritanical, privileged white bourgeois notion of gender roles onto my innocent daughter by dressing her in pink.

Many of our friends had waited to find out the gender of their children until the actual delivery, but I didn't understand the romance in that. Maybe because I was terrified of all that I was going to be worrying about during labor, and the gender of the child was only going to register a tiny blip on the graph of Major Things Going On, like, say, a human being coming out of my body and what that was going to do to my own anatomy. By finding out the gender several months before the delivery I felt that I could experience the excitement without simultaneously having to deal with the blinding pain of having the lower half of my body ripped in half.

In preparation for our ultrasound I drank almost a half gallon of water, like they told me to, and then tried not to think about the urge to go pee for two straight hours. No one will ever be able to explain to me why this is a good idea, because even on a normal day when I had not drunk enough water to drown a hippo, all I could think about was the next time I'd get to go to the bathroom. Almost like a fourteen-year-old boy thinks about sex.

But a full bladder aids in getting an accurate scan, so I did what I could, and by the time we drove to the clinic and signed in, I could feel my bladder touching my back teeth. I had to close my eyes and breathe rhythmically, my legs crossed firmly to dam the flood, and when I finally reclined on the table and the doctor touched my swollen abdomen with that cold piece of machinery I almost started crying in pain. That is, until I saw my baby's feet.

Both Jon and I had been silently worried in the weeks headed up to the ultrasound because I hadn't felt any movement in my abdomen, except for gas, indigestion, and occasional conversations with the Holy Ghost. Most of the pregnant women I had talked to said they had felt movement as early as the fifteenth week. But here I was in my fifth month not feeling anything, and I wouldn't have been surprised if the ultrasound technician scanned my belly only to find a gigantic lump of fatty deposits, or maybe a few lost tennis balls.

But immediately we saw the baby moving almost violently in the womb, and I realized that every movement the baby had been making was being absorbed entirely by the placenta. The baby did several flips while the technician tried to take measurements and then every few minutes would flash a foot at the screen, almost as if to say, Have you seen my feet yet? I'm not sure you've seen my feet. So here's this one! And look! I have another one, too!

And then, in what was one of the most memorable moments of the pregnancy, the ultrasound technician pointed to an unrecognizable shadow on the monitor and said, "See that cheeseburger? That means it's a girl."

And then he circled her cheeseburger for emphasis.

Jon had been holding my hand to give me strength to hold my pee, but right then he let go and cupped his tear-stained face. "You have a very important job," he said, looking at me with the eyes I had fallen in love with. "You're going to have to teach our daughter about her cheeseburger."

I'm pretty sure the technician permanently altered the position of the placenta because later that day I could feel the baby's every movement for hours. And the sensation didn't feel all "fluttery," a word every piece of literature I'd read had used to describe what it would feel like when the baby kicked around. When my baby girl moved it was more of a bump and a thud, almost as if she were head-butting me in anger.

It took over an hour of her kicking for me to recognize that she was moving, and that it wasn't just another bout of uncomfortable gas maneuvering its way through my lower abdomen *again*. Everything in that part of my body was constantly changing shape, and so basic functions like digestion had to rewire their usual transit maps on an hourly basis. This meant that I had gas every single second of every single day. I remember one episode of a popular sitcom where four women are sitting around a table at lunch, and the character who is eight months pregnant farts out loud in the middle of the conversation. All three other women are appalled and disgusted—how dare someone fart in public, let alone within twenty feet of their Manolo Blahniks—but the pregnant one just shrugs and says that she's pregnant and can't help it. I know someone else watching that show was probably thinking that the fart was just another one of those things exaggerated for comedic effect, that a pregnant woman could hold her wind if she really wanted to. I am here to tell you that that scene was perhaps the most realistic scene in the history of television.

A week after the ultrasound Jon and I attended a live show at a bar in downtown Salt Lake City. It was only the second concert we'd been to since I'd been pregnant, a significant decrease in the usual number of live shows we like to see. And after this particular experience, I couldn't see myself attending another live show while my body was being ransacked for nutrients by the human being growing inside. I very much wanted to be the punk rock pregnant woman who wasn't going to let the changes in her body dictate what activities she could and could not participate in, but I was done pretending to be hardcore. I had way too much sleeping I needed to get done. For future reference, I put together a small list of reasons why I will never again go to a concert while pregnant:

1. Alcohol: While it's never necessary to consume alcohol to enjoy a
   live show, alcohol consumption can always *help* a live show, if only
   by making you unaware of the humanity around you. By nature
   of being pregnant, a pregnant woman should not participate in
   alcohol consumption, and is usually the only person in the room

who is neither drunk nor stoned. This makes the pregnant woman feel like she is the only one not in on the joke, or at least that every other person in the room is excruciatingly annoying. Plus, the smell of alcohol on everyone else's breath is almost as sexy as a poopy diaper.

2. Standing for extended periods of time: By the time we walked out of the show, Jon and I figured we'd been standing for over four hours straight. I couldn't feel six of my toes, and every ounce of blood in my body was stuck in my ankles. At one point while waiting for the band to take the stage, I could no longer endure the feeling of blood pooling in my calves, so I sat down on the sticky concrete floor. Two separate people spilled beer on my head as they tried to maneuver around me, cursing me in the process for ruining a perfectly good pint.

3. Cigarette smoke: This is such a divisive issue, but nothing is more infuriating than coming home from a live show smelling like someone else's carcinogenic, respiratory crud. Although it is illegal to smoke in public places in Utah, it is still legal to smoke in bars and venues, and everyone does it with a religious fervor usually reserved for sacred temple ceremonies. I hate breathing second-hand smoke, and I'm guessing my baby doesn't like breathing it, either. Smokers will tell me to avoid bars and shows if I don't like it, and that is what I plan to do. However, I don't think it's necessarily fair to have to give up seeing the show of a band I like (whether or not I'm pregnant) because someone else cannot go an hour without a hit. And now I will go back and hide under my rock.

4. Pretentious rock stars: There is something about being pregnant that puts life into startling perspective, and in those first five and

a half months I called my mother at least once a week to say I'm sorry, please forgive me for everything I've ever done. Never before had I had such a sense of what is and isn't important, and people like the bassist of the band we saw just need to grow up. I'd never seen someone so upset to have to play a bass line. I'm willing to bet that *his* toes weren't swollen to the size of a large grapefruit.

At 2:34 AM one morning I scurried blurry-eyed into the bathroom for my nightly pee break, the first in what was usually three to four stumbling trips past bulky furniture and menacing doorways that seemed to grab my pinky toes every time I walked by. I'd grown to appreciate those nocturnal pee runs as they were the only time the baby wasn't sitting directly on top of my bladder, and I could pee more than a half-thimble at a time. Often during the day I would call out from the bathroom to Jon in the other room, "Do you hear this?" and he'd get quiet enough to witness the four-minute drip-drip drizzle as I performed somersaults and handstands on the toilet in an effort to maneuver my bladder into peeing position.

I'd been warned that this would happen, that there would come a time in my pregnancy when I wouldn't be able to empty my bladder in one go. But no one ever told me it would happen so early, or that I wouldn't be able to empty my bladder in fifteen goes. During that 2:34 A.M. morning pee run I was seized with an almost paralyzing panic, a sickening realization that I was at *that* point in my pregnancy, a week before my third trimester, the point when my body would start to become so unbearable that the lesser of two evils was going through labor.

I was so disappointed that The Belly did not feel like a natural exten-sion of my body, and that was perhaps the biggest misconception I had about what it would be like to be pregnant. There was nothing natural about The Belly. It felt like an alien object had been implanted haphaz-ardly into my abdomen, perhaps a basketball inflated with twenty pounds of loose gravel, and it was constantly shifting its weight from organ to organ.

Did I mention that this twenty-pound basketball had legs and arms and an annoying habit of trying to get my attention every night at 11:30 P.M. by poking her toes into my bladder? It was cute the first time it happened, for the first fifteen minutes. But two constant weeks of twinkle toes had me concerned that she suffered attention-deficit/hyperactivity disorder, or worse yet, that she took after her father and was up late typing angry letters to Mormon senators.

I knew that her raging activity would be gone eventually, that I'd miss the hourly thumping and nudging and bumping up against my spleen. But I was having a hard time concentrating on basic conversa-tions, on simple activities like counting out change at the grocery store, on eking out the tiniest bit of pee after a full ten minutes of sitting on the toilet with my leg behind my head.

And that is where having a husband came in handy.

Although Jon and I hadn't yet enrolled in birthing classes, which everyone said would empower us with pain management techniques and teach us how to work together to get the bulging baby here, we were already pretty good at being each other's partner.

Anyone who is married or has ever been married knows that it takes both people to make a marriage work. For instance, one person has to drive the car while the other person hangs out the window with a bat to demolish the neighbors' mailboxes. Jon is better at driving, and I have much more anger to work through than he does, so we're comfortable with our respective roles.

Additionally, he's very good at conversational distraction and can keep my mother occupied while I steal toilet paper out of her bathroom. We're always looking for ways to work together to save money.

When it came to the pregnancy, however, we had to work extra hard to figure out ways to balance out the burden. Even though he couldn't carry the baby or have his ankles swell on command, he somehow managed to will his body into experiencing some of the symptoms of pregnancy, like nausea, abdominal bloating, and frequent grumpiness. Every pregnant woman should have a partner who can moan in pain with her *and mean it*. Although he was still so skinny that I could use his hip bones to slice raw meat, there was nothing that said "I love you" more than Jon standing sideways in front of the bathroom mirror bemoaning the fact that this baby was making his ass look bigger.

We also figured out a technique to make it easier for me to empty my bladder, a position called The Ten and Two, where the left leg sticks out toward the ten on the clock, and the right leg sticks out toward the two. Once the legs were in place I leaned over forward as far as possible, and the bladder opened up and spilled pee like manna from heaven.

If there was ever any doubt as to whether Jon and I were meant to be partners, that doubt would be squashed entirely by our graceful mastery of The Ten and Two peeing procedure, which went something like this:

Jon, standing near the bathroom door, shouted, "Are you doing The Ten and Two?"

Me, strategically positioned on the toilet, left leg toward ten, right

leg toward two, leaning so far forward I was nearly kissing the bathroom floor, "I'M DOING THE TEN AND TWO."

Jon, in the middle of performing a toe-touch and handstand, continued shouting encouragement, "Ten! Two! Ten! Two!"

Me, holding my breath and pushing so hard that every vein in my
forehead was about to explode, screamed through clenched teeth,
"TEN . . . TWO . . . TEN . . . TWO."

After hearing me pee for more than two seconds Jon finally cheered,
"Goooooooo Heather!"

And then we'd repeat the whole process every fifteen minutes for the
next eight hours.

I was convinced that we didn't even need to sign up for birthing
classes because we could get that baby here through The Ten and Two
alone.

CHAPTER FOUR

Dressing Like a Concubine in Humpty Dumpty's Harem

*I*t was only a matter of time before the little indentation in the middle of my belly erupted in a volcanic burst of nubbly flesh, and all at once I was sporting the dreaded pregnant belly button. I named him Fred.

I couldn't have been more horrified at the thought of a small plug jutting out of my flesh like a gigantic third nipple, even though the top of my belly button had already formed a frowny awning in the months leading up to this dreaded development, perfect for protecting the bottom half of my belly from inclement weather and sunburn.

As I watched it inch outward, suddenly parallel with and then breaking free of the curve of my growing abdomen, I couldn't help but feel completely powerless. Having already given up control of my bladder, appetite, and complexion, I thought that my belly button was *mine*, something from my old body that I could hold on to. I considered it deep enough that I wouldn't have to worry about what would happen during pregnancy, but I had a little less than three months to go and if it continued protruding at that rate, it was going to look like I'd had a third breast surgically implanted at the waistline by the time I went into labor.

The belly button revolt was just one of the things I thought wouldn't happen to me. In fact, the list of things I thought I would never have to endure is so embarrassingly long that I ought to be publicly mauled by all the women who had been warning me the whole time that the worst was yet to come. At the top of that list was "I will never waddle," because I thought that I would have way too much dignity to be caught walking like a drunk monkey in public. But first I started teetering and then that teetering turned into a full-on waddle that became so exaggerated that I was constantly losing my balance and ramming my massive weight into cars as I walked through parking lots. Once I even left a dent, but I didn't leave my name or number because what would I have said? "Tell your insurance you got sideswiped by an ENORMOUS PREGNANT LADY."

I also thought that I couldn't possibly become a more clumsy numbskull. But there I was in the third trimester wholly incapable of uttering a complete, coherent sentence, one that didn't cause Jon to look over at me in total confusion, like, who *are* you? I couldn't think of the right words to use for anything, and one night after dinner, even though I knew that I wanted to store the leftovers in a Tupperware container, I repeatedly told Jon to put the lasagna in the tussle-wob-naters.

"The *what?*" he kept asking.

"THE TUSSLE-WOB-NATERS!" And the more I repeated it, the more it sounded right.

And then there was that one time I accidentally threw my sunglasses into a seven-foot-high Dumpster, because they were in the same hand I was using to toss away a bag of dog poop. I actually thought I might try to climb inside to retrieve them, but I knew that if Jon found out that I was rapelling down the inside of a garbage receptacle in my six-months-pregnant state, he'd kill me before the bacteria would. And then that afternoon I fell down the basement stairs as he listened helplessly three rooms away, and the pain in his worried face when he came to pick me up off the floor was worse than the bruise on my left thigh and the near fracture in my left foot.

So I tried to take the stairs a little more slowly, tried to cut my waddle from a five-foot to a three-foot radius of destruction, started thinking through words and syllables before my vocabulary turned into a string of cindenipherable won cents. And when it came to that traitorous belly button, well, let's just say we had a bulk-sized container of duct tape in the basement.

I had read about all these symptoms, that they might crop up, but it seemed like I was inviting the woes of pregnancy onto my body *just by reading about them beforehand.* It was as if reading about a symptom made it manifest. For instance, it wasn't until after I had read about "pink toothbrush" that my gums started to bleed when I brushed my teeth before going to bed, and I'd always been a pretty vigorous tooth brusher. Give me a new toothbrush and I can whittle the thing down to nothing but a shabby nubbin of its former self within three days, using nothing but my teeth and gums. But the moment I *read* about the sensitivity of a pregnant woman's gums my mouth swelled with so much blood I looked like the Vampire Lestat after a hard night of hard partying in the Castro.

So imagine my dread when I read about hemorrhoids.

Almost all of the literature I'd been reading, books and essays that listed symptoms month by month, had saved mention of hemorrhoids until the sixth and seventh months. They do this probably because it's not until this time in the pregnancy that the body becomes so unwieldy that it actually becomes necessary to push or physically urge things along when using the bathroom. I think these books are doing a huge disservice to the unsuspecting pregnant woman, someone like me, who might think that hemorrhoids, much like cancer and twins, happen to other people. I think they should warn women much earlier, like when we're in kindergarten, because I could have used that kind of time to gear up for this.

Having battled constipation my entire life, I fancy myself a veritable expert in the avoidance of hemorrhoids as I have fine-tuned the ability to push just enough and never too much. But I should have realized that the rules for hemorrhoids, just like the rules for everything else, dramatically changed for my pregnant body wherein the mere act of *thinking* about not pushing could produce an anal irritation the size of a small watermelon. So when the thinking about not pushing turned into trying not to push turned into IF I DON'T PUSH I'LL NEVER PEE AGAIN, the resulting weapon of mass destruction that sprouted on my ass could have taken out most of northern Utah if it had landed in the wrong hands.

Again, I'm not talking about a normal hemorrhoid; I'm talking about a pregnant hemorrhoid, and it was exactly like the pregnant pimple and pregnant stretch mark in that it was not a mere manifestation of pregnancy. It was an actual alien life form exploiting the gestational nature of my body to try and grow a body of its own. The pregnant hemorrhoid wanted to take over the world and was physically capable of growing fingers and toes. If left unchecked it would have mapped out a Middle East peace plan and given control of the West Bank to itself.

• • • •

One morning in the middle of my third trimester I woke up only to find that I had outgrown yet another piece of clothing, a pair of pants I'd bought three months earlier that was four sizes bigger than the pants in my nonpregnant wardrobe. That left me with exactly four items of clothing that I could actually wear, including a pair of my husband's plaid pajama bottoms which I am embarrassed to report were frequently worn in public during daylight hours.

I knew it was time to invest in maternity wear. I couldn't continue to deny the fact that my belly had transformed into such an awkward shape that the only thing that was going to fit any longer was an industrial-sized canvas drop cloth. But I hadn't ever been a big clothes shopper and found it hard to justify buying a pair of pants that I would only be able to wear for two months when the average life span of a pair of pants in my wardrobe was longer than the series run of *Law and Order*. I would have rather spent fifty dollars on a really good dinner at a Thai restaurant than on a sturdy, name-brand pair of pants, even though I knew the pair of pants would last 700,000 times longer than a serving of massaman curry. I knew it made no sense, but food tasted better than clothing, and that's where my priorities were.

Because I had yet to purchase any maternity clothes, I was still wearing T-shirts and sweaters from The Old Life, and this annoyed the more conservative members of my family to no end. I think they saw my exposed pregnant belly as some sort of scarlet letter, that I was announcing to the world in a broad stroke of flesh that I had had sex. Sadly, the only thing I was announcing to the world by wearing a T-shirt that barely covered the top of my belly was that I had gained two pounds yesterday.

I was also supposed to be setting some sort of an example to my nieces and nephews about modesty and whatnot, and baring my midsection in public was, I suppose, evidence that I was a coke-snorting whore for hire whose evil flesh would burn at the second coming of Jesus Christ. The last thing my family should have been worried about was what my clothes were saying to their children, which was, if they listened really closely, "Dressing in clothes that are too small for your body like Aunt Heather does makes you look COMPLETELY FUCKING RIDICULOUS." They should have been much more concerned with how I planned to dispose of the bodies of their children after I sacrificed them at the altar of Satan, which had been my master plan ever since I'd left the church and started listening to KISS.

I eventually gave in and started wearing those atrocious pup tents that they try to pass off as clothing, the shirts that flare with a full fifteen-foot circumference at the waist. And I even surrendered and bought a pair of elastic-bellied denim trousers that did nothing but make me look like a cheap concubine in Humpty Dumpty's harem. But I didn't wear the maternity clothes in front of my family, if only to force them to get over my bare belly and all the sinful sex that got it there in the first place. I should point out that since Jon and I were married, our sinful sex was state sanctioned, which in Utah means approved by God. So my bare belly was, for all intents and purposes, a righteous, God-fearing belly with a place reserved in heaven for itself and all its polygamist wives.

Throughout my pregnancy I'd been asked two questions consistently more than any other, the first one being: now that you're no longer Mormon, how are you going to teach your child the difference between right and wrong? My response to this one, if I didn't first start speaking in tongues or crying blood, was, I don't know, I think a few billion people in this world have done it before, it's not like I'll be breaking new ground.

And the second question was: you have a dishwasher to sterilize bottles, don't you? Which I took not as a question but more of a serious warning, that if I didn't have a dishwasher I might kill my baby with an unsterilized bottle and spend the rest of eternity in a fiery Hell with other evil mothers who never owned dishwashers.

When we bought our house at the beginning of my pregnancy, we knew that we would one day have to remodel the kitchen. All of the appliances were twenty years old, and the room wasn't even wired for a dishwasher or disposal. When a large enough number of other parents convinced us that the eternal and spiritual consequences of not owning a dishwasher far outweighed the fact that our 32-inch tall countertops prohibited us from owning one, we threw up our hands and bought one anyway, thinking that we would just cut a hole in the countertop and shove the dishwasher up against the wall.

That plan proved impossible, and we were faced with a decision between taking back the dishwasher, the key to the survival of our baby, or taking apart the whole kitchen. Let's just forget for a moment that I couldn't bend over at the waist, and that the biggest home improvement project Jon and I had ever participated in involved $29.99 IKEA lighting, and that during that project I came within a millimeter of accidentally drilling a hole in his butt. If we forget those two crucial FACTS OF LIFE and just concentrate on the idea that we started a kitchen remodel in the middle of winter in Utah when the average temperature hovers just below freezing, all without the aid of an experienced contractor, then you'll see how reasonable I am when I say that our firstborn child will drink from sterilized bottles for the rest of her life and, by God, *she will be thankful for it.*

The remodel involved the complete destruction of the existing kitchen, which included the removal of three layers of flooring, demolition of a wall of built-in cabinetry, and hacking into over twelve feet of eighty-year-old lathe and plaster. While it would have been totally possible to demolish the whole room by letting me waddle around the kitchen for a few hours, taking out chunks of wall with my mammoth thighs, we opted instead for crowbars and sledgehammers which weren't in danger of going into early labor.

And when I say "we" I am totally misleading you, because I really had nothing to do with the demolition. I may have plucked a few staples from the wood floors here and there, and you'd never in your life have seen a more enthusiastic, pregnant cheerleader, but 121 square feet of Smurf-blue kitchen was smitten and sent to Jesus through the hands of one very tired father-to-be.

While I had prepared myself for life without a kitchen sink or stove or oven, I had no idea the actual physical toll the project would take on my already ravaged and swollen body, or that I would become so desperate as to end up on my sliver-infested knees promising the Mormon God that if he would just make it end already I would stop telling my sister's children that sacrament bread is laced with arsenic.

After we took apart the kitchen, we were faced with a decision between tiling the kitchen floor or prepping the wood for refinishing, and because choosing the easy way out would have been too logical or easy, we opted for the latter, a decision on par with deciding to remodel the kitchen when I was eight months pregnant:

Dumb.

Our floors were not just covered in a layer of dust and dirt, no. They were coated with a quarter-inch crust of an asphaltlike adhesive and three layers of cardboard. In order to remove that crust we had to spread a toxic chemical adhesive remover in small squares across the floor and then scrape, inch-by-inch, centimeter-by-centimeter, over and over again. The first night of The Armstrong Wood Floor Prepping Disaster yielded a whopping one-square-foot area of scraped wood flooring. By the end of that night—after almost five hours of continuous scraping, after my arms and fingers could scrape no more, after I had tried to will the scraper across the floor with the sheer power of my mind alone—I sat huddled in a lumpy, pregnant mass in the corner of the kitchen, lead-paint respirator pulled up around my forehead, tears pouring down my dusty cheeks.

Jon, bless his heart, not only had to deal with his own set of scraping, but also the inconsolable idiot in the corner wearing his carpenter pants, the waistline of which hit me in the armpits, because I wasn't willing to sacrifice any of my pregnant pants to the toxic jaws of this project. Scraping and sobbing continued in this manner into the second night, after which a whole three feet of flooring was uncovered. It was on this second night that both of our hands started to bleed and the dog, high on chemical fumes, started barking in Russian. In a delirious moment before we fell into bed that second night I halfheartedly suggested that we leave a small square of solvent on the floor overnight, just to see what would happen, even though the directions on the side of the can say DO NOT LEAVE OVERNIGHT UNDER ANY CIRCUM-

STANCES. When we woke the next morning we found that the solvent had turned the asphalt adhesive crust into butter, and that instead of five more days of scraping we were going to be able to wipe everything off in a matter of hours. Because my hormones were so out of whack I cried for an hour over the fact that I hadn't thought of trying this sooner.

This bipolar relationship with the wood floors continued the following day when I waited over eight hours for the refinisher to show up, a small Greek man who knew about three words of English: yes, no, and Tuesday, which he thought meant Thursday. And even though it took him two days more than he said it would take to complete his job, I was happy to be done with that portion of the project because it allowed me to spend a few days concentrating not on the kitchen, but on ways in which I could dislodge tiny little feet from my ribcage and drink a glass of water without getting heartburn.

When I finally did see the refinished floors I had to be physically restrained from dropping to my knees and licking their shiny goodness. It's just that small victories like that one were what was going to get me through the next seven weeks of pregnancy. I was already so uncomfortable in my bigness that I constantly felt as if my diaphragm was sitting in my throat, and I couldn't maneuver the baby's feet out from under my lungs. No amount of coaxing or pushing or thumping could get her to extract her toes from my third rib. And with as many weeks as I had to go, the baby was going to double in size, which basically meant that by the end of it her feet would be sticking up my esophagus and poking out my mouth, and I'd look as if I'd just swallowed an 8-pound baby.

On the official last day of The Armstrong Kitchen Remodeling Disaster we spent several hours patching a hole in the ceiling and filling in tiny divots in the walls left as presents from the three blond kids who installed the new cabinetry. I think they might have been distracted by my belly, because all three of them couldn't stop staring at it. And I didn't understand this, because Utah is the Pregnant Belly Capital of the World. There is no other city in the world that is home to more pregnant bellies. And then I realized that they were probably glaring at the nakedness of the belly and its distinct absence of Heavenly Underwear, and were probably secretly praying for the welfare of my unborn, innocent child about to be born to a non-Heavenly-Underwear-wearing mother. I could see their point.

Once the holes were spackled and sanded Jon and I made a celebratory trip to the grocery store to buy our first box of dishwashing detergent, and after paying cash for a giant box of Cascade I said to the cashier, "You're witnessing my first adult purchase of Cascade." Because she needed to know.

And she just looked at me blankly, unmoved, and mumbled, "I'm honored." But I knew she was lying. She had no idea of the significance of the occasion, that starting that night I would be able to sterilize baby bottles, and all of the depraved sins I had committed in my life would be forgiven.

The morning after Christmas Jon and I woke to over a foot of snow on the ground and to a house with a temperature hovering at about fifty-two degrees. Salt Lake City was in the beginning stages of a snow dump that would last almost two straight days and leave nearly 90,000 people without power.

My belly was usually very good at generating its own heat, and had on several occasions nearly singed off Jon's leg hair in the middle of the night. But that morning even my belly was cold, so we headed twenty minutes north of Salt Lake to take cover at my mother-in-law's house. Halfway through the day, however, she lost power as well, and so we headed back home that evening to a freezing house, rooms full of Pier 1 scented candles, and several minutes of heated poker playing. Both Jon and I grew up in a religious culture that disdains "face cards" as tools of the devil, and the only thing we had to bet with were M&M's candies that never made it from the bag to the poker table because my mouth got in the way.

We were among the very fortunate who had our power restored within twenty hours, but by the time the storm was over we had to deal with no Internet service and a driveway covered in over three feet of snow.

And then our twenty-seven-year-old hot-water heater kind of stopped working.

And then the guy from Sears who showed up to install the new hot-water heater that totally wasn't in the budget said that he couldn't install the new hot-water heater because of some code or permit relating to the furnace and how carbon monoxide was most likely leaking out of the chimney and slowly killing us in our sleep, and that to fix the whole death-in-our-sleep thing would cost us the college fund of our second child, the college fund for our first child having already been spent on plumbing the new kitchen.

And then Our New Dishwasher started making weird noises, noises that just aren't supposed to be made by a new dishwasher, noises you'd likely hear coming from a rotting, diseased rhinoceros as it flails its gigantic limbs in a last gasping yelp for life.

And then the guys who were supposed to pick up the old refrigerator smoked too much pot and said they couldn't pick up the old refrigerator, and I was forced to figure out a way to make a twenty-five-year-old refrigerator look a little more *cozy* as it had become a permanent fixture in the living room.

And while I was totally ready to scream and cry and wield my belly in wholly lethal and illegal ways, I was tremendously blessed to have a husband who could look at it all—after two straight days of shoveling snow, snow he'd only ever accuse of being glorious and beautiful—and smile and hold my hand and tell me *Heather, it's going to be okay.* And there was nothing in this world more magnificent than the way he said my name.

I thought that when I finally made it to the thirty-sixth week, the point after which they say the baby can make a safe appearance at any time, that I would feel calm and peaceful with what was about to happen to me, because many pregnant women in their ninth month seem to radiate an almost superhuman serenity, an impenetrable resolve and acceptance of their fate, like they are walking to the guillotine feeling nothing but happiness at the prospect of meeting their maker.

I did not feel an ounce of this calm. What had forever been an abstract concept, something that would happen *later,* was going to materialize and become a very real and realistic reality in less than four weeks. I was scared shitless, even more shitless than my usual shitlessness. And when you consider the standard I'd already set for shitlessness, this new level of shitlessness was perhaps a level of shitlessness the world had never before seen.

And it's not that I hadn't read about labor or didn't know what was going to happen to me—I was very aware of how labor works and what would happen after labor and how my nipples would feel like they were going to harden into steel bolts and fall off my chest. I'd witnessed two live births and watched in slow motion, Technicolor, wide-angle focus, the slicing inhumanity of an episiotomy. I'd asked strangers at the grocery store how they handled their first labors and endured endless half hours of baby stories on TLC involving perky women in plaid who saw no problem with having their wheelchair-bound grandmother rolled into the delivery room at the exact moment their vagina exploded with new, screaming life.

If there were two things I'd learned through my extensive study they were 1) labor is by nature a total unknown, and there was no possible way to determine what my personal experience would be like, and 2) if anyone decided to roll in my wheelchair-bound granny while my naked, sprawling vagina was pushing out a hairy, flat skull, I would personally hunt them down and tear their face off. My husband had been instructed that no grannies in wheelchairs were allowed anywhere near my delivery room. He had also been instructed that the use of sports-related metaphors to get me through contractions, such as "We're rounding third base!" or "It's the bottom of the ninth and all bases are loaded!" were grounds for immediate divorce if not death.

I think the reason I was so scared was because the whole thing seemed so unpredictable, and I have a very hard time being put in situations in which I am not in absolute control. Labor would involve the will of a wholly separate human being inside my body, a human being with the DNA of her mother and father, which basically meant I'd be dealing with the most stubborn personality that ever walked the Earth. She'd also have to make it through the birth canal with her shoulders and feet, a combination of my shoulders and her father's feet, which basically meant the average of wide and wider, and huge and huger. The only comforting, predictable factor of this labor was the idea that if she did get stuck, someone could just reach up in there, grab hold of her fully grown unibrow, and yank her into the light.

When Jon and I went to the doctor during the thirty-seventh week we learned that my belly had grown over three inches in less than fourteen days. It was encouraging news, as my belly had surprisingly measured below average for most of my pregnancy, and it seemed that this child had decided to save all her weight gain and growth for the last few weeks. I'm not sure there are words to describe just how uncomfortable it was to suddenly be three inches wider at the waist, and my doctor, sensing my noticeable discomfort, kind of rolled his eyes and said, "You haven't seen anything yet. The next few weeks will be the worst part of your pregnancy." I had never wanted to take up violence against a human being so fiercely in my entire life. No man, not even Doctor Jesus Christ, should ever try to convince a woman in her ninth month of pregnancy that he knows anything at all about what it's like to be pregnant. Just go ahead and shut up, you uterus-less clod.

Although the last couple of months had been extraordinarily uncomfortable, I would take the third trimester any day over the first thirteen weeks of pregnancy. But this didn't mean I wasn't going to go ahead and complain. In fact, the number of things to complain about in the third trimester overwhelmingly swamped the number of things about the first trimester, even though I could smell shampoo without taking a shower in my own vomit, and that alone made the last few months infinitely more bearable.

The worst part about the third trimester was my inability to sleep. I've always been an expert sleeper, almost Olympian in my skill to ease into unconsciousness within moments of hitting a horizontal surface, and have been known to sleep in bursts longer than the average life span of a large canine. But during the last few months of pregnancy I averaged about twenty minutes of solid sleep at a time, and this was due entirely to that horribly unnecessary force of nature known as gravity. Whenever I fell asleep on my left side, the weight of my body would crush my shoulder and thigh, forcing me to roll over to my right side. But where I'd once been able to roll over while still unconscious, I was suddenly forced awake involuntarily and had to physically maneuver my body into another position, usually through means of a crowbar, forklift, or a team of three to four muscular contractors trained in heavy lifting. This left-to-right-side maneuvering continued throughout the night so that by the time the alarm sounded in the morning, I'd have changed positions no less than four hundred times, leaving Jon bruised, without covers, and reminiscing about how much less energy it took to demolish three layers of linoleum than to push his wife over in the middle of the night.

I was also under the impression that everyone else in the world was pregnant, men and children included, and when I saw anyone bump their stomach into a solid surface I wanted to make sure that their baby was okay. I couldn't watch more than thirty seconds of a football game, because there were over twenty babies on that field at any given time, all in danger of being tackled and stomped. By the fourth play of the game I'd be in tears, having just seen six or seven babies smooshed into the Astroturf, appalled that these men could just run around bumping into each other without one concern for the babies in their bellies.

While watching a commercial where a gigantic man belly flops into a pool, my whole body seized and I immediately called Jon at work to ask WHY DOES NO ONE LOVE THE BABIES?! And for the remainder of the day I walked around feeling like I had done the actual belly flopping, my whole chest stinging from the impact.

Another inconvenient side effect of having a six-pound critter fighting for space in my belly was being constantly reunited with the taste and texture of things I'd just eaten. Everything caused heartburn, including water, ice cubes, and air. If I ate a handful of Tums, I'd burp Tums for the next three hours. There were nights when I'd lie awake for hours at a time, left-to-right-side maneuvering, stifling monster burps of food I'd eaten over the span of three days. A horizontal esophagus seemed to exacerbate the heartburn, so while I was trying to relax and sleep, a chunk of the bagel I'd eaten that morning was dancing on the back of my tongue with the red onion from lunch. Chuck was constantly smelling my breath and licking my face, searching for bits of the burrito I'd eaten last week.

I never could have comprehended how magical it was to be a ripe pregnant woman, belly widening inches per day, grumpy and irritable from sleep deprivation, burping acidic salsa into my dog's face. Don't let anyone ever tell you that this isn't an exquisitely beautiful experience.

CHAPTER FIVE

Labor to the Tune of Janet Jackson's Nipple

O n one of my final visits to the doctor we found out that I was
dilated to a "one plus some" (the actual medical term he used)
and 70 percent effaced. I had no idea what that meant, so he explained
it like this: let's just say that there's this thing that has to open up to the
size of a large bagel before the baby can move down the birth canal.
We're talking about a steroid-injected bagel full of carbohydrates, the
ones that count for two full meals' worth of calories. A big, big bagel.
And when that thing gets to be the size of a bagel, that is when the baby
comes out. That morning, though, it was only the size of a small Chee-
rio, which meant that I probably wouldn't go into labor for two more
years.

For a few days I'd been experiencing false labor. I knew it was false
because every seven or eight minutes I would turn to Jon and say excit-
edly, "My lower back hurts!" And he would in turn say, "That's awesome!" Come on. I wouldn't be uttering any decipherable words or
giving Jon any impression that what I was feeling was in any way awesome if it had been real labor. I hadn't given Jon too much in the way

of instructions or rules as to how to coach me through labor, except that he not get within a foot of my face with his own face. I imagined that my sense of personal space would become especially pronounced during contractions, and I didn't want to be held responsible if I bit off his nose.

I mentioned the false labor to his mother one night as we were driving her to a small town in northern Utah, and she immediately perked up. "Don't you DARE have that baby in this car!" she demanded. "I don't have my good scissors!" Even if she had only had her *bad* scissors I'm pretty sure she could have delivered the baby. Jon's mother is an incredibly talented woman, and she's constantly blurting out little insane snippets of wisdom that would sound rude or invasive if they came out of anyone else's mouth. But because she's the one who's saying it, I never take it personally or seriously.

"Cover up that belly!" she warned me toward the end of my second trimester just as my stomach had grown too big for my wardrobe. "That baby is going to catch a cold and come out diseased!" She has six children of her own. This probably happened to at least one of them.

Another time she told me, "You know, the reason you're so uncomfortable is because of all that working out you're doing! Those stomach muscles are restricting that baby!" These observations were followed by a sigh and an almost inaudible mumble about "you crazy kids," and then she sent us home with a quilt she'd made in less than two days and leftover potato casserole. I'm constantly thanking Jon for being born to her because I saw the first few seasons of *The Sopranos* and I know the risks involved with inheriting mothers-in-law.

The more I got to know her the more I understood some of my husband's more idiosyncratic personality traits, the most adorable of which was his habit of suddenly blurting out something that made no sense and had no context. We could be sitting in the car in silence, driving down the freeway, when out of nowhere he would say something like, "Junior Wixom had trouble doing that." He was either continuing a conversation he was having with someone not in the car or completing a thought he had started in 1988, but I'd have no idea who or what Junior Wixom was or what he had trouble doing. And when I looked at him like, *you do realize that you just said that out loud, right?*, he always had this great way of connecting what he'd just blurted out with something totally relevant, like, "Junior Wixom had trouble doing that, and I think you're really beautiful." And with that sort of connection he could talk about Junior Wixom and the trouble with doing that all he damn well pleased.

I had every inclination to believe that this child would be born with the same blurting out disease, much like her cousin, who once announced to a car full of unsuspecting adults, "My mom has fur on her bottom!" I was actually looking forward to the years of hilarity our child would provide just by virtue of being her father's daughter and her grandmother's granddaughter, and it will not surprise me when she tells her first grade teacher that the reason she can't complete her homework is because she caught a cold in the womb and came out diseased.

By week 39 I had not given birth, although every member of my immediate family and every member of my extended family, all eighty-seven of them, called my house to ask me about it. That wasn't at all annoying.

I was beginning to think that the sac holding the baby was made of an impenetrable material, a special blend of steel, Teflon, and vacuum-sealed plastic. My sister had five kids and her water never broke, and my mother carried me for an entire four weeks after I was due, and her water never broke. So I'd come to terms with the fact that my water wasn't going to break, but I was worried about what was going to happen in the delivery room when my doctor realized that the standard hook they use to break a woman's water just wasn't going to work on me. Isn't that one of the last things a woman wants to hear when she is sprawled naked on the birthing table? BRING ME A BIGGER HOOK.

During a late-night birthing class we got to take a look at the water-breaking hook, along with the catheter and IV bag they hook up to the woman when she's giving birth. We'd been attending a birthing class being given by the hospital where I'd be delivering the baby, and when we learned about all the equipment, including the epidural needle and heartbeat monitor they attach to the baby's head *inside the womb*, I realized that the whole purpose of the class was to scare the living shit out of expectant parents. They were constantly showing us videos of women screaming during labor or saying things like, "THAT doesn't look like a baby!"

The blond woman teaching the class had never had a baby, and she openly scolded me when I shouted out, "Cigars!" in response to the question, "What should you bring with you to the hospital?" I'm not sure what I was supposed to have said, the Holy Scriptures? A clean set of Heavenly Underwear? Because those are two very important items in a birthing plan, right up there with tequila and porn, if you ask me. I think I may have crossed the line during a discussion about the pros and cons of breastfeeding when I suggested that one of the advantages of formula feeding was being able to get back to my rock-and-roll life-style. You've never seen a more frightened group of pregnant women, many of them terrified that their child would one day encounter my child and be introduced to the evils of coffee and MTV.

The classes were causing me to have strange dreams, one in particular where Al Roker was demonstrating proper breastfeeding techniques to me and the rest of my classmates. He had enormous nipples and was handling them with an almost unlawful carelessness, just swinging them around and pinching them and mushing them like little red meat patties. He made sure to warn us that we shouldn't try this at home, not yet anyway, because persistent nipple stimulation had been known to induce labor. And I knew he specifically mentioned that part because I had just read about the whole nipple stimulation technique, that there are some doctors who recommend that a pregnant woman past her due date try twiddling her nipples for up to three hours at a time.

Three whole hours of nipple twiddling.

I can hardly imagine doing anything for three whole hours. I did see that three-hour movie about the hobbit people, but I wouldn't describe that experience as watching a movie for three hours. I'd describe it as more of a three-hour countdown until I could pee again.

Friday, 30 January, 7:00 PM: For the fourteen days prior to this evening I had tried every possible labor-inducing technique documented in pregnant folklore to get this baby here including but not limited to:

1. Furious stair running, which in my nine-months-pregnant condition was more of a furious stair *waddling*

2. Hour-long walks with the dog

3. Praying

4. Seducing my husband more frequently than should be legal for a swollen human incubator who had worn nothing but elastic-waist pajama bottoms in public for the last four months.

I even thought about twiddling my nipples.

We had heard about a local Italian restaurant that served Pregnant Pizza, a specialty dish that had sent at least five pregnant women into labor according to a local newspaper. Of course, local newspapers in Utah do things like feature spreads on polygamy that read like glowing advertisements for the fanatical offshoots of the Mormon Church, but I was desperate and willing to try anything short of agreeing to let my daughter be married off at the age of fourteen to a sixty-year-old who thinks he's been ordained by God.

I ordered the Pregnant Pizza, which was just a 144-square-inch pool of garlic, and as an appetizer ate a dish that contained over one hundred cloves of roasted garlic. By the time we left the restaurant I'd consumed so much garlic that I expected to give birth to a daughter who would poop garlic for the first thirteen years of her life.

Saturday, 8:00 AM: Jon gave birth to his "baby."

Saturday, 9:00 AM: I felt nothing. I hadn't farted or belched or felt any gastrointestinal movement, although it smelled like a garlic bomb had been detonated in our bedroom.

Saturday, 1:00 PM: Chuck took a poop in the backyard and it smelled like garlic.

Sunday, 6:00 PM: Consigned to the reality that I would never give birth to my garlic baby, we settled into the garlic haze of the bedroom to watch the Super Bowl. Perhaps it was the garlic hangover or maybe because we're reasonable adults, but we rewound Janet Jackson's half-time boob malfunction only once. Jon asked with barely any interest, "Was that her boob?" and I answered, "I think so." I had bigger boobs to worry about.

Sunday, 6:30 PM: I started feeling lower back pain in throbbing sixty-second cycles. The pain was noticeable enough that Jon broke out his watch and started timing the intervals. One interval was eight minutes. The next was five minutes. Some were fifteen minutes, but there was definitely a start and stop to the pain.

Sunday, 9:30 PM: After three consecutive hours of back pain I suddenly realized that I needed to poop! Pooping was glorious! Except! I spent the next hour in the bathroom passing My Garlic Poop, and it left me with gigantic garlic hemorrhoids. And then the random back pain completely stopped.

Sunday, 9:30 PM–11:30 PM: Jon spent two hours trying to reconcile the fact that he wasted three precious hours of his life timing poop labor.

Monday, 9:00 AM: My doctor told me that I was dilated to a three, meaning my cervix had opened to three centimeters, and that I was in perfect condition to be induced. I didn't want to be induced, not with my garlic hemorrhoids, but he said that he was going to be on vacation for most of the week and that I may go into labor when he wasn't in town. That would mean that some other doctor who had never seen me before would deliver my baby, some other doctor who might just like to give episiotomies for the hell of it, and I wasn't ready to relinquish my intact vagina to a stranger.

He asked us if we'd like to do it today. Today? You mean, this day? *The day that is this one?*

Jon and I looked at each other like, was there anything we wanted to get done before the birth of the baby? Aside from 1) a honeymoon to Paris and 2) extensive experimentation with hard drugs, I couldn't think of anything, so we both shouted, "YES!" Normally we would have emphasized our enthusiasm with a colorful word or two, but my doctor was very Mormon, and I didn't want to upset the man who would be holding sharp instruments near my private parts.

The doctor made a call to the hospital and they said we should go home, pack a bag, take a shower, and wait for a call that should come by 11 AM, the earliest that they would have a free room.

Monday, 11:00 AM: We had showered. We had packed. We had called the family including my mother, The Avon World Sales Leader, who was canceling a flight to LA so that she could be here for the birth. We were staring at the phone. The phone wasn't ringing.

Monday, 11:05 AM: Ring, damn phone! RING! Why wasn't it ringing?

Monday, 11:07 AM: I asked Jon to check and make sure the phone was working.

Monday, 11:08 AM: Jon assured me that the phone was indeed working.

Monday, 11:09 AM: The phone wasn't ringing. I began to hyperventilate.

Monday, 11:15 AM: The phone still wasn't ringing. I began to pace the floor and contemplate the horrible words I was going to spray paint on the front door of the hospital.

Monday, 12:00 PM: I called the hospital to let them know that they were torturing me and that I was going to sue. They said that the woman who was giving birth in the room that they were going to give to me just needed to push the baby out. Oh, WAS THAT ALL. They said the room would definitely be ready in about four hours, and that amount of time sounded longer to me than my entire pregnancy.

Monday, 12:15 PM: We threw everything into the truck, including the dog, and headed to my mother-in-law's house where Chuck would be staying for the next five days. We made sure that we noticed how cold it was outside, how cold and gray and dirty, so that when we told our daughter about the day she was born we could begin by saying, "It was a cold and gray and dirty day in February." That just sounded like something a parent would say. We were going to be parents!

Monday, 1:30 PM: HOLY SHIT WE WERE GOING TO BE PARENTS.

I'd changed my mind. I didn't want to give birth. I voiced my concern out loud. Jon's mother, a woman who had given birth six times, gave me a look that said I pretty much needed to shut up. I shut up.

Monday, 2:00 PM: Back pain again. I guessed that I would need to go poop in about three hours.

Monday, 3:00 PM: I was still having back pain. I convinced Jon to call the hospital to check on our room even though it had only been three hours. The hospital said that the room would definitely be ready by 4:30 and that in order to get the room we would need to be there at exactly 4:30. I suggested we leave immediately even though the hospital was only fifteen minutes away. Jon was reluctant to indulge my irrational behavior, but we prepared to leave anyway and gave instructions to his mother concerning the dog: no potato chips, no raw meat, and she needed to make him work for treats.

Monday, 3:15 PM: We left Jon's mom's house. Chuck received his first potato chip.

Monday, 3:30 PM: Jon was driving slowly. We tried to enjoy our last car ride as a childless couple. It was the last car ride of our Old Life. I felt like I was going to throw up.

Monday, 4:00 PM: We arrived at the hospital and carried all of our luggage up to the fourth floor. I wanted to tell every single person I saw that I was going to have a baby. I had to physically restrain myself from singing in the elevator.

Monday, 4:05 PM: The nurses sitting behind the desk in the labor and delivery area regretted to inform us that they had given away our room just two minutes ago to a woman delivering triplets prematurely. As if that was any harder than what I was doing? Three was only two more than one, and that was not very many. I asked if we could share the room. They said no.

Monday, 4:07 PM: Despite Jon's best efforts to comfort me I warned the nurses behind the desk that the Avon World Sales Leader had canceled a flight to LA just so that she could be here when I delivered my baby, and that if they knew what was best for them they would give me a room and not upset the Avon World Sales Leader. Accordingly, they told me to go wait in the waiting room and that a room should definitely open up within the next hour. And then they rolled their eyes.

Monday, 4:10 PM: The waiting room was filled with hundreds of little kids. Maybe not hundreds, but it felt like hundreds with all the bratty screaming. Jon and I realized that we'd made the huge mistake of trying to have this baby in Utah, the Baby Making Capital of America. It could possibly be the Baby Making Capital of the World, but there is probably a third world nation out there whose inhabitants have had no education on contraception, and that third world nation may have one or two more babies than Utah. We started to realize that we might not ever get a room.

Monday, 5:30 PM: Still no room, but my back pain had become really uncomfortable. So uncomfortable that I had to get up and walk around. My doctor had just delivered another woman's baby and visited us in the waiting room. He regretted to inform us that they had yet again given away our room to another woman and that we might have to go home and come back the following day. I nearly clawed his eyes out.

I mentioned my back pain, and then he asked, "How far apart are the pains?"

"Four minutes," I answered, which I guess in doctor-speak meant I'M IN LABOR.

Monday, 6:00 PM: WE GOT A ROOM!

Monday, 6:10 PM: I changed into the dreaded hospital gown and was introduced to my nurse, who was four feet tall and had a gray mustache covering her upper lip. I couldn't stop staring at the mustache. It was just so hairy. And thick. And I wondered if Jon noticed her mustache. How could he not notice her mustache? The nurse delivering my baby had a mustache!

Monday, 7:00 PM: I spent the hour giving The Mustache my entire oral history per hospital regulations. So many questions! None of their business! Just get this started already! GAHHH! She had a mustache!

Monday, 7:10 PM: Mustache hooked me up to a contraction monitor and a Pitocin drip, the hormone used to get the contractions really going. We turned on the television to CNN *Headline News,* just to have some background noise. And hey! There was Janet Jackson's nipple!

Monday, 7:30 PM: I'd been on the lowest dose of Pitocin for about twenty minutes and my contractions were already three minutes apart and lasting sixty seconds each. These were contractions? These?? These here?? NO PROBLEM! I could totally handle this. This was easy! They were uncomfortable, yes, but to someone who had been constipated her whole life THESE WERE NOTHING! Hey! There was Janet Jackson's nipple again!

Monday, 8:00 PM: I was dilated to a four. My mother, my sister, and my stepfather showed up. My mother, the Avon World Sales Leader, was dressed in her best business attire. She looked like she had shown up to fire Donald Trump. My bare vagina was lying right there on the hospital bed, and my mother was perfectly pressed. I hoped her suit had been Scotchgarded.

We all watched Janet Jackson's nipple. Again.

Monday, 9:00 PM: I was dilated to a five. The contractions were becoming a little more intense but they were still manageable. Jon's sister, who happened to be a labor and delivery nurse at another hospital, showed up. Mustache informed us that her shift had ended and that another nurse would be taking care of us. What? No more mustache? But I wanted my baby to be delivered by The Mustache! Come back, Mustache!

Monday, 9:30 PM: New nurse arrived and didn't have a mustache. In fact, she was perfectly harmless and boring. Nurses should be required to have mustaches.

Monday, 9:45 PM: Jon's sister was showing Jon how to help me breathe. The contractions were intense enough that I really needed his help. Together we pushed through the pain: hew, hew, hew, hew heeeeeeeee! Hew, hew, hew, hew heeeeeeeee! Hew, hew, hew, hew heeeeeeeee!

Jon was wonderful. He was right beside me holding my hand. We couldn't believe how easy this was! Bring on the baby! And look! There was Janet Jackson's nipple again!

Monday, 10:00 PM: "Did you hear that?"

"What?"

"That."

"What that?"

"That!"

"WHAT THAT?"

"That popping sound."

"What popping sound?"

"You didn't hear that pop?"

"What pop?"

"That pop! I felt it in the back of my mouth."

"I didn't hear any pop."

Monday, 10:02 PM: My water gushed all over the hospital bed.

Monday, 10:03 PM: "Oh . . . THAT pop."

Monday, 10:04 PM: I ran to the bathroom so that the nurse with no mustache could clean up the bed. While I was in the bathroom I had my first contraction post-water-breaking and it was curiously unlike all the pre-water-breaking contractions: REALLY FUCKING AWFUL.

Monday, 10:06 PM: I returned to the hospital bed and told Jon that the pain was getting a lot worse. In the middle of my sentence another contraction hit, and I almost bit off my tongue.

Monday, 10:15 PM: AWFUL AWFUL AWFUL. Contractions that were three minutes apart and lasting only sixty seconds were all of a sudden ten seconds apart and lasting ninety seconds. The nurse realized that the combination of the Pitocin and my water breaking had thrown my body into a transitional state—what is supposed to happen when someone is dilated between eight and ten centimeters—even though I was only dilated to a six. I started to shake violently, and my body was covered in chills. I could barely see straight. The nurse turned the Pitocin off.

And there was Janet Jackson's nipple, my constant, calming companion.

Monday, 10:25 PM: I was on the verge of vomiting all over the bed. The pain couldn't possibly get worse than this. During one of the ten-second breaks I asked all the women in the room if it would get any worse than this. They all looked at each other silently. No one would answer me.

It was going to get worse? It could not possibly get worse. Worse than that was dead. There couldn't possibly be a worse pain in the world. It felt like someone was trying to twist the top half of my body off my lower half, like I was a plastic Coke bottle.

Monday, 10:30 PM: I was going to die. Labor was going to kill me. Jon was trying to help me breathe, but my body's pain-coping mechanism was forcing me to hold my breath. I was only getting ten seconds of a break between contractions, and I wasn't getting enough air.

IT WAS REALLY AWFUL.

Monday, 10:35 PM: I was officially writhing. There was actual writhing going on. Unabashed writhing.

Monday, 10:40 PM: Jon forced me to look into his eyes and breathe: "Hew, hew, hew, hew heeeeeeeee! Hew, hew, hew, hew heeeeeeeee! Hew, hew, hew, hew GET ME THE EPIDURAL!"

Monday, 10:45 PM: The anesthesiologist showed up. Talk about service!

Somehow, in my awful, writhing state, I noticed that he was wall-eyed. His left eye was looking at Jon; his right eye was looking at me. It only confused me more. I had to tell him that I understood what he was going to do and all I could think about was how brutal his childhood must have been, having those wall eyes and all. Children are cruel. I knew, I was about to have one.

Monday, 10:50 PM: I signed the epidural release form. He turned me on my side so that he could stick the needle in my back. I realized that one of his eyes was looking at my back, the other one was probably looking at the ceiling.

I was in the middle of a contraction that was about to crush my body. Jon was holding both my hands and looking me straight in the eyes.

"You can get through this," he assured me. I had to hold still so that the anesthesiologist could stick the needle in the right place. Holding still was the hardest thing I had ever done.

I felt a small prick in my back and my leg flexed involuntarily. The anesthesiologist said that he was done. I didn't believe him. He couldn't possibly be done. It was supposed to hurt and I was supposed to freak out about the needle! He was done?

Why had I been so scared? WHY DID I WASTE WEEKS AND WEEKS OF MY LIFE WORRYING ABOUT THE EPIDURAL NEEDLE! GIVE ME THOSE WEEKS BACK!

Monday, 11:00 PM: The epidural had taken effect. It was the best feeling I had ever felt in my life. I wanted to smoke a joint. I started to sing. My mother and sister started laughing. I asked Jon if we could name the baby Epidural Armstrong.

I was so happy!

Monday, 11:30 PM: Did I mention how happy I was? They should sell epidurals on the street. I would buy a hundred of them and give them to my friends.

Tuesday, 12:00 AM: Still happy! Everyone was talking and laughing and joking. And guess what felt good? The epidural!

Tuesday, 1:00 AM: I was dilated to a nine and I felt no pain. At that point we had seen the replay of Janet Jackson's nipple over one hundred times.

Tuesday, 2:30 AM: I was dilated to a ten and it was time to start pushing. I didn't feel like pushing but they assured me that it was time.

Jon stood on my right side; his sister stood on my left side. They held my knees to my chest and the nurse told me to take a deep breath and push.

"Huh?"

"Push."

"Push where?"

"Just push."

"How do I push?"

Tuesday, 2:35 AM: I thought I was pushing, but I didn't really know if I was pushing. It didn't feel like pushing. It just felt like I was holding my breath. Jon's sister and the nurse exchanged a silent glance like, *this* is going to take a while. I wanted to tell them that there was no way that this "pushing" thing was going to get this baby here. This pushing thing was stupid. There had to be a better way.

Tuesday, 3:00 AM: Still pushing. I was pushing for thirty seconds every two minutes. Pushing was more tiring than any of the workouts I did during pregnancy. Pushing was hard. I looked into Jon's eyes each time I pushed and noticed that he was unconsciously pushing with me. He was beginning to get light-headed.

Tuesday, 3:15 AM: Jon almost passed out from pushing so hard. I warned him, "IF YOU WANT TO LIVE TO SEE TOMORROW, YOU WILL NOT PASS OUT."

Tuesday, 3:20 AM: Still pushing. My mom and my sister shrieked simultaneously. They could see the baby's head. Apparently the baby had hair! The nurse asked me if I wanted the overhead mirror to see what was going on. NO, I DIDN'T WANT TO SEE WHAT WAS GOING ON. ARE YOU PEOPLE CRAZY?

Tuesday, 3:30 AM: My doctor arrived and stood at the end of the hospital bed to assess my progress, and I could see the reflection of the carnage of my vagina in his glasses. HORROR!

HORROR!

Tuesday, 3:40 AM: I wanted to ask my doctor to take off his glasses so that I wouldn't be confronted with my own reflection, but at that point the baby's head was crowning and I could feel my body stretching around her skull. Why could I feel that? That felt weird.

Tuesday, 3:45 AM: OUCH. BABY'S HEAD. BURN. BURNING. OUCH. OUCH. OUCH.

Tuesday, 3:50 AM: The doctor said something to the nurse at that point, something about how he thought he wasn't going to have to, but now he had no choice, and he reached for something, and Jon whipped his head around to look at me, and then I felt a snip and a release of pressure. Thank God I hadn't agreed to the overhead mirror.

Tuesday, 3:55 AM: The doctor made a second snip. I felt everything. The burning had subsided, but I could still feel the contour of the baby's head. I couldn't describe this feeling as anything but weird. My mom and my sister were literally jumping up and down at this point, both jabbering on about all the hair on the baby's head.

Tuesday, 3:58 AM: I felt the baby's head come out of my body, and then I felt her shoulders. OH MY GOD IT WAS WEIRD. She was twisting as she came out, and I could feel everything. I felt her arms. Then her belly. Then her legs.

Tuesday, 3:59 AM: My mother, the Avon World Sales Leader, started screaming. My sister was crying. Jon was more lovely than I had ever seen him in my life. The doctor dropped this thing on my stomach, and HOLY SHIT! IT WAS A BABY! I honestly didn't know what he was going to pull out of me, perhaps an abandoned tire iron, or maybe a bag of potatoes? I felt so much relief that it was human.

Tuesday, 4:00 AM: Jon cut the cord. The baby was whimpering quietly. They wiped her down and placed her immediately on my chest, her right arm stretched out toward my face. She and I looked at each other directly. Jon leaned down, placed his left hand on my head, his right hand on the baby's back. It was the most defining moment of my life.

We made a family.

CHAPTER SIX

You Have to Feed the Baby . . . Through Your Boobs

We named the baby Leta Elise Armstrong. She was named after my mother's sister, Leta Kay, who died when she was five months old. Leta rhymes with Rita and pita and, of course, Dorito. At birth she weighed seven pounds, ten ounces, and measured twenty inches long. Her official birthday was 02/03/04, which should make it very easy to fill out forms when she applies for a mortgage.

She had long toes she got from her mama, but otherwise she looked exactly like her father.

Some women say that their babies look like an opossum, gerbil, or other type of lovable rodent. But ours? Ours looked like a frog.

The first seven days of having a newborn baby in our home were the most difficult, most humbling string of incoherent hours of my life. I'd never been more tired or more weepy or more terrified or more joyous. I couldn't do anything but focus on making it hour to hour. I'd had really low expectations for labor, meaning I thought it was going to be a horrific, gory experience, and I know that it is for many women, but it was because of those low expectations that I could, seven days later, look back and say that labor had been a somewhat pleasant, perfectly manageable process. The lesson to take from this is, of course, to aim low in life and be thrilled when the worst doesn't happen. I was a new mom, and look at all that wisdom!

What hadn't been manageable, however, was the inhumane aftermath of labor that I hadn't heard anyone talk about. Just when I thought things couldn't get any worse—worse than the level two vaginal tear and subsequent stitches, the hemorrhoids of such mythological proportions that the nurses at the hospital were surely going to tell stories about them for the rest of their careers, the bleeding, the abdominal contractions and cramps, the fatigue—I developed a urinary tract infection and also became unbearably constipated.

Seven prescription drug bottles sat on my nightstand, among them pain relievers, antibiotics, prenatal vitamins for breastfeeding, and a huge container of stool softener. I was under the impression that stool softener was supposed to soften the stool, and maybe for normal people who pooped normally, stool softener may have done what it was supposed to do. But I'd never pooped normally, remember? And all the pushing I did during labor confused my entire system so that the stool softener did nothing but sit there pooling like freshly poured concrete in the lower half of my body. A few days after returning from the hospital I spent over four hours in the bathroom, and all the relaxation techniques I'd learned for labor became laughably inept as I screamed and screamed for mercy.

So I started drinking prune juice like it was water, and immediately it had a very interesting effect on the baby, who had finally taken to breastfeeding. Everything I'd ever read about breastfeeding had to have been written by a man with no tits, because everything said that as long as the baby was in the right position it wouldn't hurt to breastfeed. THAT WAS A LIE.

The only way to describe it to a man is to suggest that he lay out his naked penis on a chopping block, place a manual stapler on the sacred helmet head, and bang in a couple hundred staples. The first two staples might hurt a little, but after that it just becomes numb, right? And by the eighty-eighth staple you're like, AREN'T YOU FULL YET? But then the comparison really fails because a man doesn't have two penises, and after stapling the first boob the baby moves on to the *other* boob and the happy stapling begins ALL OVER AGAIN.

I decided many years ago that when I eventually had kids I would try my hardest to breastfeed them. I knew it would be something I would have to work at because my sister, whose boobs are far bigger and seemingly more life-giving than mine, had such difficulty trying to breastfeed each of her five kids that the longest she was ever able to feed any of them via the breast was one month. And it wasn't that she didn't try very, very hard. It's just that her milk had the consistency and nourishment of water, and her kids were left starving after each feeding. So she switched to formula, and now she and all her five healthy children are going straight to hell.

During my pregnancy I looked forward to breastfeeding and the possibility of bonding with my baby while simultaneously providing her with gobs of antibodies and tailor-made nutrients. I didn't need to be convinced that breast is best, and every time I picked up a book to read more about the process of breastfeeding I had to wade through at least two to three chapters devoted specifically to convincing me that women who use formula are terrorists. Apparently, everything that has ever gone wrong in the world can be traced back to some evil woman who fed her baby a man-made imitation of breast milk via a plastic nipple. The literature on breastfeeding can sometimes be obnoxiously fanatical—there is one book that actually says that needing a good night's sleep is a myth perpetrated by the bottle feeders of the world!—and if we took it to its logical conclusion we wouldn't be looking for Osama bin Laden in the war on terrorism. We would be looking for his mother and her stockpile of deadly Similac and Enfamil.

I don't personally think that my sister is a bad person because she decided to feed her babies from a bottle—my sister is a bad person for entirely unrelated reasons involving aerosol hairspray. I have a lot of respect for her and the difficult decision she made for herself and for her children, and after my own intense experience of wielding my torpedo boobs, I can say with a tiny bit of authority that breastfeeding is not easy. They will tell you that it is easy. They will say it's good for you, it's good for your baby, and it's easy! And they will be lying to you. SHOVING A BLUNT PENCIL INTO YOUR EYE IS EASY, TOO, so there is no merit to that claim, and you shouldn't believe them.

I think back to those first few days of breastfeeding, and I'm overcome with agony because I know that there is some new mother out there right now who had her baby hours ago, and she is trying to get that baby to attach, and that baby is just madly gumming at her bruised chest. I am so, so sorry, new mom. In case they didn't tell you, breastfeeding isn't easy.

Nipples learn quickly, however, and after a few days of successful feeding they become immune to the stapling, and the piercing pain turns into dull, uncomfortable throbbing. Some feedings are worse than other feedings, and in Leta's case, the worst feedings were the ones in which she held conversations with my breast. And I'm talking pages of dialogue, single-spaced. Usually these conversations were upsetting, because she'd scrunch up her nose and throw her knee into my other breast, all while bobbing her head back and forth to emphasize her point. And that wasn't particularly fun because when her head bobbed my nipple bobbed, and NIPPLES WEREN'T MADE TO BOB.

Perhaps the hardest thing about breastfeeding, which also happened to be the hardest thing about new parenthood, was nighttime when her sleep schedule often interfered with the agenda of my breasts. When she didn't wake up for a few hours to eat, my boobs, normally emptied throughout the day, started to fill up with milk. Consequently, I'd lie on my back completely awake as my breasts hardened like mud in the afternoon sun. Sometimes it was so bad that my boobs were literally exploding, and the only relief I could get was in a handheld breast pump that creaked as I tried frantically to elicit milk from my nipples.

One night I sat in the dark, nipples creaking, my hand cranking the pump like a well in the desert, and nothing would come out of my boob. I cried quietly for a half hour, mumbling to myself, *my boob doesn't work!* But Jon could only take so much, and he finally sat up in bed and put his hand on my right arm. "Put down the breast pump and go to bed," he said. "Your boob totally works."

I was feeding about every two and a half hours, and since I'd started drinking gallons of prune juice the baby was pooping every two and a half minutes. That's an exaggeration, sure, but you should have seen these poops. Jon and I were totally fascinated with the color and texture, as if she were some sort of Picasso weaving neon orange creations into her diapers. I was very jealous of her ability to poop so regularly and with such artistic flare, but I was also elated that her body seemed to be thriving. Every time I heard her fill her pants I got so excited that I wanted to frame the dirty diaper and hang it on the refrigerator.

Every time I changed her diaper I was overcome with a sense of fulfillment, and I felt that way in the most un-hip, earnest way possible. My life before Leta felt like it had happened decades ago even though she was only a week old, and I never knew I could love someone or something so intensely or so achingly. I'd spend several hours a day just listening to her breathe. I couldn't stop smelling her neck or sticking her little frog feet in my mouth. She was the most perfect creation in the world, the most innocent bundle of coos and yawns and mumbles, and my heart broke every time she focused on my face.

The weekend after Leta was born we picked up Chuck from my mother-in-law's house where he had been staying since we left for the hospital five days earlier. It was the first time I'd left the house since returning home from the hospital, and I was certain it would be the last time I would see the outside of my own home for at least the next six years.

It took us over an hour to prepare to leave the house, stuffing everything we thought we might need into one tiny diaper bag, including shaving cream, conditioner, three medical journals, two rolls of toilet paper, all seven of my prescription drug medications, and no less than seven changes of clothes for the baby, all for what would end up being two hours away from home. But we needed all those things, *just in case*! After that experience I wondered why I would ever want to leave my house again.

I had remembered my thirty-five-pound mutt as being a somewhat lithe, gentle creature, very tiny in his thirty-five-pound frame, but when

I opened the door and he came running to greet me, I was confronted with an enormous, unrecognizable monster. WHO HAD FUR. *FUR!* His size seemed odd, yes, but it was his fur that made me rub my eyes to make sure I wasn't seeing things, I was just so used to dealing with a skin-covered baby. It didn't help that Grandma's house served as a five-day all-you-can-eat buffet of treats and pig's ears and what else, Grandma? Popcorn. And? And toast. And? And apples. And? Okay, fine, and bacon grease.

We introduced Leta to Chuck in Grandma's living room, a some-what neutral space where Chuck wouldn't have the instinct to protect his property. And from the rabid tail-wagging and drooling you could tell that Chuck thought she was some sort of enormous treat swaddled in yummy pink velvet. He couldn't sniff her head or face enough, and he kept looking at Jon and me like, this is for me? The whole thing? All of it?

In the days that followed he behaved remarkably well in the presence of the baby, especially considering the fact that our daily outings to the dog park came to an abrupt halt. If anything, he'd become more at-tached to me and less likely to leave the room when I entered it. He was fascinated with Leta's high-pitched coos, and whenever she made a sud-den noise he'd sit up straight, stick his ears to the sky, and look at me like, you better not be hurting that treat!

In the mid-eighties there was a song about not having to take your clothes off to have a good time, that the good time could be had drink-ing cherry wine, and its video ran in regular rotation on *Friday Night Videos*. Somewhere in my basement I have a VHS tape with that video and the one for "Papa Don't Preach" and that Peter Cetera song from one of the *Karate Kid* movies. I blame my parents for that serious lapse in good taste because they never taught me to look outside of popular radio and television for music, and they only smiled with pride when they found out that I had made a cassette filled entirely with "We Are the World," taped off the radio, over and over and over again. Even before I became a parent I knew that I was going to make sure that my children grew up listening to Bob Dylan and Miles Davis. I'd teach them about Jimi Hendrix and the broad cultural significance of Milli Vanilli.

But I remember being so excited about weekends as a kid because it meant I'd get to see that video, and in my adult life I hadn't experienced quite the same enthusiasm for Friday nights, not until I brought home a baby and she locked me in my bedroom. Friday nights suddenly became very special because they signaled a two-day vacation from being the only diaper-changer. Jon would get to stay home from work for the weekend, and we'd resume our tag team dynamic, one that involved headlocks and body slams and elaborate eye makeup.

When Jon went back to work after only five days of paternity leave, I felt like I was running a marathon that didn't have an end. Leta was initially a very good baby; she didn't cry very much during those first few weeks and was content to sit and look around, occasionally grunting and pooping, but I'd never been so nervous or frantic in my entire life. Was her poop the right color? Was she breathing too fast? Her feet were blue! Were her eyes supposed to cross like that?

To help Jon understand what it was like to stay at home alone, I put together a small list of things I'd learned in the short time I'd been with our daughter:

1. A good day was defined entirely by personal hygiene. Brushing my teeth = pretty good day. Brushing my teeth + brushing my hair = I was doing really good. Brushing my teeth + brushing my hair + taking a shower = WORLD DOMINATION. I believed that if I could get all the way to putting on mascara that I'd be magnificent enough to create my own planet and populate it with bears.

2. Leta came equipped with an internal altimeter that could detect the exact moment I wanted to sit down while holding her. It was so sensitive that it set off an alarm when my knees started to bend, so I couldn't even *think* about sitting down when trying to soothe her. Sometimes we performed an awkward polka where I'd bend my knees, and just when she'd start to fuss I'd straighten right back up, over and over again, and it sounded like someone in the neighborhood had set their car alarm to "infant despair": WAH! . . . WAH! . . . WAH! . . . WAH!

3. Sleep deprivation was going to kill me. Leta knew how to poop, she knew how to eat, SHE HAD TO KNOW WHAT TIME IT WAS, FOR CRYING OUT LOUD. At 2:00 AM every morning she looked up at me with huge Armstrong eyes as if to say, hey, where's the party? I was under the impression that there was a party going on. Take me to the party.

4. Leta didn't like *American Idol*, and that was a serious crisis as we never missed a single episode. How could she possibly call herself an Armstrong if she didn't consume lowbrow American pop culture with the same hunger she approached mama's breasts? Was I going to have to start acting like I actually had taste?

5. Breastfeeding got much, much easier because my nipples had become so numb and callused that I could have safely nursed a full-

grown crocodile without feeling the slightest pinch. People had always told me that I was going to be surprised at how big my boobs would get when my milk finally came in, but I was in no way prepared for how fucking ridiculous they would look. My cleavage was so high that I could rest my chin on my right boob, and I could shoot rockets at low-flying satellites out of my avocado-hard nipples.

6. Baby poop smelled like buttered popcorn.

To celebrate that first Friday night back together, I ran around the house bending over and touching my toes, over and over again, and then tied and retied my shoes with effortless speed. The things you take for granted when you're not gestating life. I was a mad and mean bending-over machine and seriously contemplated spending the majority of my weekend bumping my belly into walls and countertops JUST BECAUSE I COULD.

Instead, Jon and I spent those next three days holed up in our bedroom, what we affectionately referred to as The Cave. It had become the center of our home, where we ate, where we slept, and where we would have pooped if we'd worn diapers and had two fumbling, gangly parents to wipe our bottoms. I never knew that I could be so satisfied to sit and watch another human being for hours at a time, and there was barely a moment that weekend when I didn't gaze at The Biological Wonder and think to myself, *how the hell did that come out of my vagina?*

In addition to staring at Leta like two drooling, lobotomized idiots, we did a lot of scratching, stretching, catnapping, and watching an obnoxious amount of reality television. It's amazing just how much television I didn't watch during the week when I was trying to take care of a baby. In fact, it's amazing just how much of everything I neglected, things as basic as plucking my eyebrows, which had grown so unruly that they had eaten half of my forehead.

And then on that Sunday afternoon we decided that it was time to face my new worst fear, worse than my fear of heights or natural disasters, worse even than my fear of biscuit containers that go POP when you unravel their cardboard exteriors, and that fear was the fear of taking Leta to a public place. I was frightened of the diseases that lurked in public places, viruses that could have wreaked havoc on the immune system of a fourteen-day-old baby, but I was more scared of being that woman with the screaming baby that I'd so often wanted to choke or beat with a wooden club. I had to keep reminding myself that the worst thing that could happen would be that she would start crying and either Jon or I would pick her up and comfort her while the other stuffed groceries into the shopping cart. It wasn't like Leta would all of a sudden stand up in her car seat, pull out a machine gun, and open fire on unsuspecting grocery shoppers.

But I needed to come to terms with the possibility of some grumpy single person shooting me a disapproving look as I bounced a fussy baby in one arm while reaching for a gallon of milk with the other, as if a fussy baby has no business being in a public place. I was once that grumpy single person, and I feel her pain, the pain of sleeping more than eight hours a night, the pain of eating a warm meal with two hands, the pain of chugging two double vodka martinis without fear of poisoning another human being. And I want to say to the grumpy, single me of several years ago—the grumpy, single me who kept up with her eyebrows and had her nails professionally manicured every

two weeks—I want to say, *you just wait!* And then I want to choke her
and beat her with a wooden club.

At Leta's first appointment with the pediatrician we learned that she'd
gained twenty-one ounces in the fourteen days since we'd left the hospital, which meant mama's milk made mouths happy! I knew she'd put
on some weight because there were times when she'd wake up for the
first of four times during the night and I'd think that her head had gotten bigger in the two hours she'd been asleep. But twenty-one ounces?
In two weeks? That either meant she was going to be valedictorian of
her high school because she was developing at such an advanced rate,
or that she'd weigh over six hundred pounds by the time she was five
years old.

Venturing out to the doctor's office, however, did not prove as easy
as her weight gain. Neither Jon nor I had slept more than two consecutive hours since bringing the baby home, and when I couldn't get the
car seat to fit into the car . . . in the snow . . . as the snow was falling on
my baby's face . . . as the snow froze my hands . . . the hands that
couldn't get the back door to shut . . . the door that was warped from
all the wet snow . . . after yelling at the dog because he wouldn't get
back into the house . . . after comforting the dog because he was so
displaced . . . I stood there crying in the snow. Bawling in the snow.
Screaming in the snow. Rattling off a string of four-letter words. In the
snow.

I'd never cursed so much in my life.

I finally gave up and stomped back into the house, picked up the
wireless phone, took it back outside, and called Jon to have him walk

me through the process of putting the car seat into the car. But once I heard his voice all I could do was stand there and scream, gigantic tears pouring from my eyes and freezing on the side of my face. Somehow he managed to calm me down enough that I noticed I had the goddamn thing in backwards, and once I turned the seat around it clicked in automatically, without any effort whatsoever.

I thanked him, told him I loved him, and apologized for exposing his daughter to such profanity. And then I climbed into the driver's side of the truck, turned on the heat, and cried for another five minutes.

There was just so much crying.

There were really good days, days when I felt strong enough to handle this job, days when I looked at the future ahead of us and got excited about the ride. On good days I could go several hours without crying.

And then there were bad days, days when I couldn't imagine leaving the house again, days when I thought that by the time I did leave the house again my hair would be past my waistline, because how could I ever get my hair cut when the baby needed to be fed every two hours? On bad days I thought I'd never be able to walk the dog again, I'd never go shopping again, I'd never see a movie in a movie theater again. On bad days I imagined growing old in a dust-covered house surrounded by hundreds of mounds of dirty laundry and piles of forty-year-old poopy diapers because I'd never again have the strength to clean my house. On bad days I cried all day long.

Jon tried to help, tried holding my head when I cried, but I was inconsolable. He always ended up walking into another room to take long, deep breaths. Sometimes he had to walk around the block to cool off his frustration. Sometimes I would wake up in the middle of the night to find him crying, and I knew it was because he was watching his wife go slowly insane.

Being a mother was the hardest thing I had ever done. It was really, really hard. It was impossible to make a single coherent decision when I was completely beholden to another creature's sleep schedule, and that creature happened to sleep in random ninety-minute blocks. It wasn't so much sadness I felt but utter delirium, and by the end of the day when we faced another night of not knowing if she was going to sleep, it was hard not to ask myself, how the hell can I do this another day?

And then the sun would come up, a full two hours after we'd tried unsuccessfully to get her back to sleep for the third or fourth time during the night. Delicate new light would flood the room, and I'd notice that her eyebrows had gotten darker overnight. Her cheeks were fuller, her thighs thicker, and she'd be wildly kicking her frog feet. She was thriving and gaining weight like a champion. And then I'd slowly get up and do it another day.

CHAPTER SEVEN

Sympathy for the World

I was always afraid that Jon was going to suck Leta's brain out of her nose when he tried to clean out her boogers with the blue rubber syringe. Clearing out someone else's nasal passages was not something I signed up for when I acted on my biological urge to procreate. Neither was the dreaded clipping of the infant fingernails. Those things served more to torture me than they helped to keep Leta de-clawed or snot free, and when Jon would gleefully reach for the infant clippers I'd have to flee the room and hide my head in the oven.

You'd think that I would have been prepared for this, having practiced for years on the dog's claws. But you haven't seen Chuck's claws up close and in person, and I'm sure that if you did you would have a completely different opinion about me and my notion of decency. I am horrified by the popping sound of the clipping and the very real possibility that I might cut him and cause him to bleed, something I have done on more than one or two or ten occasions.

When we clipped Leta's fingernails for the first time, we cut off all peripheral noise, turned on all the lights, and held our breaths until near suffocation. It took about an hour to finish all ten fingers because we would pause between each clipping to admire each and every adorable joint and knuckle in her hand. It had become a pastime in our home to dissect the DNA of all of Leta's body parts. The knuckles on her index fingers came straight from her father. Her cuticles were definitely mine. The size of her hands in general was the monstrous combination of the two families colliding.

Things were getting better only in the sense that I was becoming used to living this way. Parenthood was turning my whole body into one giant callus. Each passing day was unbelievably hard, harder than when I thought things couldn't get harder, but my crying fits slowly disintegrated into fits of eye-rolling or sighing or throwing my hands up and saying to myself, Seriously? You couldn't wait to pee until I had put the diaper ON your butt?

One thing I could not get used to was the anxiety attack that hit me every day at about 6:30 PM when I started to realize that I might not get to sleep that night. Leta's sleeping schedule was completely unpredictable despite our best efforts at establishing some sort of routine to set her clock. During the day I didn't let her take naps longer than a couple hours, and I'd listen to music or to the TV at an elevated volume to signify DAYTIME! When it was time to go to bed we gave her a warm bath and then turned off all the lights. We tried sleeping with her in between us, underneath my arm, on Jon's chest, in a bassinet beside the bed, all to varied and irregular results. She was very loud when she slept, and as her mother I heard every sound she made—every grunt, every sigh, every angry attempt to pass a stuttering fart. She'd go an average of three minutes without making a noise, and then at the end of that three-minute stretch she'd explode with noises as if to say, ha ha! Just kidding!

And it didn't really matter how many hours she'd been awake during the day. Her primary goal in life was to torture me, and she figured out that the easiest way to do that was to stay awake by any means possible. Her strategy one week was to spit out her pacifier every five or six minutes and then make loud noises until I stuck it back into her mouth. So I'd spend the hours from 10 PM until 2 AM sticking her pacifier back into her mouth. By 5 AM in the morning, after two feedings and another hour of pacifier relocation, I considered duct taping the damn thing to her face.

Dear Leta,

I am writing this letter to you here on the day that you turn one month old. I cannot possibly tell you how significant this is because I honestly didn't think I would ever make it past the first hour. Just yesterday you smiled at me for the first time. It made me cry, which isn't necessarily significant considering that your poop makes me cry, but you smiled with your mouth wide open and your eyebrows raised in delight. I had read that you might be smiling at me by the fourth week, and at the end of last week I was sweating bullets that you might not reach this milestone on time. What if you never smiled? What if we'd given birth to a smile-less baby? Could a smile-less baby get into college?

And then BOOM, you smiled all of a sudden, not once or twice but four times in a row. I spent the rest of the day breast-feeding and downloading applications for early entrance into several Ivy League schools.

To celebrate these four weeks, your father and I went out to dinner alone for the first time since you were born. I have only left the house a couple of times in the last month because this winter is one of the worst I have ever lived through, and carrying around a heavy car seat through two feet of snow is not at the top of the list of things I want to do on no hours of sleep. In fact, there is only one thing on that list: cry.

You are still too young for me to feel comfortable leaving for any extended period of time, and when we left you with my mother for just a couple of hours so that we could grab a bite of sushi I felt like I had cut off my arms and legs and could think about nothing but getting back to you. On the drive home it seemed like we caught every red light in the city, and it infuriated me to think that the city planners hadn't thought about this specific circumstance. There are mothers out there right now trying to get back to their tiny babies and they can't because of traffic lights. Which makes me believe that a mother should be consulted on every decision that's made on Earth.

The entire day after we ate sushi you were in a terrible mood, and this means that I won't be eating sushi again anytime soon. Because when you are in a bad mood the whole family suffers, including the dog whose response to your disgruntled shrieking is to jump on and off the bed, over and over again. This bed-jumping routine has become his reaction to everything you do, and to someone who isn't chronically sleep deprived it might be cute. But in the middle of the night, here in week 5 of Project Leta Doesn't Sleep, his compulsive bed jumping feels like someone is poking me in the eyeball with a toothpick.

The list of things that you do not like is relatively small and includes things such as having the light turned on suddenly in the middle of the night, or having cold lotion rubbed on your naked belly. Every night after your bath your father and I wince right before we stick your arm into your nightgown, because there is nothing so upsetting in this world as having to put one's arm into a nightgown, obviously, and we spend the next half hour dodging your wailing screams as they bounce off walls and melt the hair off our heads. When you are in the middle of an encounter with something you don't like, the last thing I should do is stick the pacifier in your mouth because you are fully capable of spitting it four feet across the room.

I've also learned not to sing you lullabies when you're upset because it seems that my singing voice is at the top of the list of Things That Make You Regret Being Born. I've tried loud singing and soft singing and somewhere in between singing, but your reaction to all of the singing is to get a pained about-to-pass-gas expression from your chin to your wrinkled forehead that says WHY ARE YOU TRYING TO KILL ME?

Message received.

This last month has been a mixed blessing for me, Leta. You have changed my life so markedly that sometimes I don't know who I am anymore. I did not know that I was capable of such strong emotions, both good and bad, and the only way I know how to deal with such emotions is to cry. You and I spend our days together on the bed listening to music on my laptop, and some of the songs I play only make things worse because they remind me of the days before you came into our lives, days when I could sleep when I wanted to, days when I was not physically chained to this house.

But I am not that person anymore. I am now your mother, and while thoughts of the future sometimes suffocate me with worry, they also make me feel so much more sympathetic to the world. In just the few short weeks that I have been a parent I feel so much closer to my own family, closer to what it means to be human. I feel like I have been let in on some secret that all other parents know, that they would have shared with me if they could have. But it's a secret that I had to learn for myself, through loving you, that the fullness of life begins and ends outside of myself. By choosing to bring you into our family I have made an irreversible commitment, and the joy of the love I feel for you is as meaningful as it is because the loss of it would break my body in two.

Love, Mama

CHAPTER EIGHT

It's All Fun and Games Until Someone Pokes Their Eye Out With a Baby

Throughout the nine months of my pregnancy Jon and I were warned constantly by other parents to enjoy sleeping while we could. Many of our friends even suggested that we stock up on sleep, as if it were something you could seal in a Ziploc bag and toss into the freezer, something you could warm up in the microwave and mix with a little creamer on the nights when the baby refused to sleep. I'd really like to smack those parents because not only was that particular piece of advice unsolicited, it also wasn't helpful at all.

You can't store sleep in your jowls for the long winter ahead, so just stop patronizing soon-to-be parents with that absurd suggestion. Just say what you mean, which is, *your life is going to be miserable, and I will take great pleasure in seeing you squirm.*

If there is one thing I would tell soon-to-be parents, one thing that no one ever took the time to tell me, one thing no book or doctor or nurse cared enough to tell me, it would be this: the longest stretch of sleep you will get in the first month of your baby's life will be four hours, and you will be very, very lucky if you can actually score four in a row. You will most likely sleep in two-hour blocks at completely random times throughout the day. The best way to deal with this torture—and it is torture, the worst torture you will have ever endured—is to realize that millions of us have been through it and are going through it right now. You have to look at it in the face and accept it, wholly and completely, with every tired limb of your body. There really is no way to prepare for this, and the only way to find any comfort is to understand that you are not alone.

After almost five weeks of living with a newborn, I'd only once slept for four hours in a row, and that was on the second night in the hospital when the nurse took the baby to the nursery for the night. My complexion was terrifying and I could have used the bags under my eyes to haul groceries, but I had to believe that living that way wouldn't cause any permanent damage to my long-term health. I mean, how many other women have lived through this, right? However, I was in danger of traumatizing my child with the massive wrinkles around my eyes, and I feared she'd grow up with the ugliest mom in the neighborhood.

When Leta was born all sorts of maternal instincts were slammed into the ON position—the instinct to protect, to nourish, to comfort. And no matter where she was sleeping or pretending to sleep, whether in our bed, on top of me, in a bassinet beside the bed, or in her crib all the way over in her own room, I had to retrain my body to sleep. My instincts were telling me that when I slept Unknown Things happened, and my body resisted the urge to fall asleep. I was unconsciously listening to the sound of her breathing or swallowing, and if those noises sounded okay then I'd listen to the sounds of the house to make sure monsters didn't crawl out of the walls to hurt her.

I had every reason to believe that those instincts would become numb with subsequent children, but Leta was my firstborn, and I had no idea how to turn it all off. She could have slept through the night, but I'd lie there awake for hours waiting for something terrible to happen. Was I torturing myself? I didn't know how not to. Perhaps the most frustrating thing about it was that I didn't know how much longer it would continue, how much longer I could go on. I didn't expect to get more than two consecutive hours of sleep for at least another couple of months, and by that time I'd be such a lunatic that surely I'd go missing for a few days until Jon found me crouched in a corner, drooling, scratching sores that didn't exist, mumbling to myself, *what was so wrong with our old life that we had to go and do THIS to it?*

For nine months I grew a human being inside my belly and then pushed it out my vagina. Afterward I fed it with my boob. Biology is so fucking weird.

I just really needed to point that out.

There wasn't an official breast person to stand by and make sure that I was doing the whole feeding thing right, but I had to assume that my boobs were working because Leta completely outgrew all of her 0–3 months clothing before she was even two months old. Her legs started to stick out of her nightgowns like a little hobo baby, and her head became huge. Gigantic. Enormous. Sometimes I'd look down when I was feeding her and it looked like I had a hairy cantaloupe attached to my boob.

I defy anyone who is breastfeeding a five-week-old baby to go a whole ten minutes without saying boob or breast. That was the only word I could get out of my mouth. It was boob this and boob that and my boobs did this today and can you believe my boobs? When I answered the phone I said, "Boob?"

I wasn't sure whether or not it would happen so soon but I finally arrived at a point where I actually liked breastfeeding. There were still moments when Leta latched on so fiercely that I was afraid she might bite off my boob (see? boob! boob! boob!), but otherwise it had become a magical, deeply moving experience. Not the type of magical that I had sparklers or smoke shooting out my nipples, but in the sense that I had this ability to comfort her instantly and that feeling was really powerful. I'd also developed a technique that didn't require I be surrounded by fifty pillows to support my arms. My goal was to be able to breastfeed and load the dishwasher simultaneously, and when that happened I planned to take my act on the road.

My mother bought me four Sears brand nursing bras that I would rotate through my wardrobe. They were the most utilitarian pieces of clothing I'd ever owned and looked as if they were designed with the shape of a four-hundred-pound communist factory worker in mind. But I swore by those Sears brand bras. They were brawesome. They were comfortable enough to sleep in, which meant I didn't ever have to wake up in a puddle of my own milk. The breast pads I wore to soak up the leaking, however, were not Sears brand and were a little less friendly than the bras themselves. They were boob-shaped maxi pads made of disposable cotton that stuck to the inside of the bra, self-adhesive side out, and I had to get used to the idea that as long as I breastfed this kid I'd have to walk around with crinkly boobs.

Crinkle, crinkle, crinkle.

Regardless of the inconvenience of the crinkling I was really glad that I'd stuck with breastfeeding. It's true what they say about the unique bond between mother and child that is facilitated by the tender intimacy of the act, and there were moments in between feedings when I looked forward to the next feeding, to feel her frog feet kick at my chest, to feel her coconut belly pressed against my own.

However, I was completely unprepared for the bone-crushing pangs of The Breastfeeding Hunger. Everyone talks about hunger during pregnancy, myself included, and that hunger is typically about specific cravings. So specific, in fact, that you shouldn't be surprised if your pregnant wife wakes you up at 3 AM asking for a Whopper from Burger King, an order of fries from McDonald's, and a Frosty from Wendy's. It would behoove you to honor these cravings as if they were orders from God, because a Frosty from Wendy's is completely different from a milk shake from McDonald's, and if you bring back a milk shake from McDonald's your baby will most likely grow up never knowing his father.

Jon had it easier than most men because my cravings were always for things we had stocked in the house. We bought bags of Nacho Cheese Doritos in bulk, and if I ever had a craving in the middle of the night he only had to go as far as the kitchen cabinet. There were moments, however, when the only thing I wanted to eat was whatever Jon had sitting on his plate, and even if he ordered the largest carton of fries on the fast-food menu he was lucky to get even two of them from the plate to his mouth successfully.

The Breastfeeding Hunger, though, is far more consuming than the Pregnancy Hunger because it isn't about specific cravings, although if the dog had been covered in chocolate I would have totally eaten him. The Breastfeeding Hunger is more about craving every kind of food. It is an equal opportunity hunger, a hunger that does not discriminate, a hunger that believes homosexuals should be allowed to marry.

Breastfeeding made me hungry all the time. Once I finished breakfast I was thinking about my midmorning snack and what it would feel like in my mouth. Toward the end of the day I'd get so hungry, so panicked in my hunger, that Jon knew better than to ask me what I wanted to eat. I DIDN'T WANT CHOICES! I WANTED FOOD! Choices take time to sort through, and last time I checked time didn't taste like anything or have any nutritional value. So I'd just open the refrigerator and start eating. Sometimes I'd forget to take off the plastic outer wrapping of whatever I was eating, but isn't that what the large intestine is for?

One night Leta was sitting contentedly in her car seat, and we decided to use that opportunity to cook an actual meal on the stove with food that wasn't packaged in a box. I prepared two full plates to carry to the dining room table—the place where childless people eat their meals, memories!—but somewhere on the ten-foot journey from the kitchen countertop to the dining room I ate everything on my plate. And I would have eaten everything on Jon's plate, too, had he not held it high above his head so that I could not reach it. It was his small way of saying HAVE SOME DIGNITY, WOMAN.

One day during Leta's seventh week of life my mother agreed to watch her for a few hours so that I could get my hair colored. I guess the word "agreed" isn't necessarily correct in the sense that my mother informed me that she would be taking my baby away from me for two hours, and I either comply or be written out of the will. Not wanting to jeopardize the lifetime supply of Skin So Soft I stand to inherit, I gave in without any argument. I'd never seen my mother so in love with another human being, and there were nights when I'd hear a noise outside and I was certain that my mother was there to kidnap the baby.

I was thrilled that my mom had become so involved in Leta's life. Family was the primary reason Jon and I moved back to Utah, and I honestly couldn't have made it through those first seven weeks without my mother's help. She single-handedly stocked Leta's entire wardrobe, and although the clothes were flashier than I would normally prefer, I didn't see the harm in having a daughter dressed like a mini Avon World Sales Leader. Plus, we could use the money we saved on baby clothes to buy more chocolate.

Leta was still too young for me to feel comfortable leaving her for any extended period of time. When I did leave her, I felt like I was cutting off my arms and legs, and I was left an armless and legless nubbin who could think about nothing but getting back to her. When I was forced to leave her, though, I trusted her with no one but my mother. She had that annoying grandmotherly ability to comfort a baby just by entering the room. I studied her to see if I could figure out how she did it, but she had no discernible technique. Was it something they taught at grandmother school? How could I enroll?

Leta would be wailing that certain baby wail that said *I am now officially possessed by the Devil,* and I'd pace and shush and sway back and forth, and the Devil inside my daughter just laughed at me. My mother, however, wielded some sort of secret Pope-like power and could cast out the demons just by picking her up. It was infuriating! And of course she did it with a wickedly smug grin on her face as if her perfect hair hadn't already made me feel incompetent for years. In those instances I wanted to threaten my mother that if she looked at me like that again her granddaughter would grow up surrounded entirely by Revlon products, which to the Avon World Sales Leader would be the equivalent of threatening to register my daughter as a Democrat.

Regardless of our occasional tensions I was really grateful for the two hours I got to spend having someone fix my embarrassing roots. While the color dried on my hair I had the almost orgasmic luxury of reading a magazine uninterrupted, and when I glanced at the table of magazines sitting next to me I almost passed out from the possibilities. Should I read an article in *Vogue* or spend the whole fifteen minutes reading *People* from front to back? Maybe I'd just look at the pictures in *Us Weekly*. THE DECISIONS WERE THRILLING.

By the end of the seventh week I figured I had the hang of this thing, this thing being my new job as mother of an almost two-month-old baby. I hadn't mastered this thing by any means, but I'd at least come to a point where I didn't panic when Jon left for his job in the morning, and I was faced with spending the next ten hours ALONE WITH A BABY. For a while it felt like he was leaving me alone with a bomb, and if I turned away from it at any point during the day it would explode and destroy the whole world. But things got better and it started to feel more like a hand grenade, and I just had to resist the urge to yank out its safety pin, which in Leta's case was picking her up when she was perfectly content to lie on her back. There was no cradling of the hand grenade in our household, because the hand grenade would look at me like *T-minus three seconds before I blow your hand off.*

There were moments during the first few days of Leta's life when I really didn't think I was cut out for this whole thing. I remember feeling very inadequate because I'd known some really stupid people who had kids, and I thought if really stupid people could do the whole kid thing, why was I having such a hard time? But look! At almost two months in I was finally gaining on the stupid people! Somehow I'd managed to go over fifty days without doing any permanent damage to myself or to the baby, and when you consider that I've always had a chronic problem with not being able to walk around walls but only straight into them, having a dent-free baby was something I could put on my resume.

I'd had other jobs in my life where I was unable to meet the standard set by stupid people. During the summer after my freshman year in college I attempted to wait tables at a very popular chain restaurant. I thought it would be an easy way to make a fair amount of money in a short period of time, and since I had just aced calculus the semester before, I thought I would have no problem taking an order for a hamburger and bringing it to someone's table. Little did I know that my mastery of differential equations would have no bearing whatsoever on my ability to fulfill a drunk Southern woman's request to bring her taters and biscuits. I had dated a really stupid guy in high school who could wait tables (he was stupid, yes, but he did have great hair), and when I quit after three days I cried at the realization that I wasn't as smart as stupid people. I was so stupid that I couldn't even bring taters.

After I graduated college I took a full-time job as a phone reservationist for an airline and had to sit with my ear pressed to a phone for eight hours a day fielding calls from the American public. I had a college degree, I thought, how hard could it be to memorize fifty airport codes? But the only thing I learned from that job was that I could only remain in a seated position for forty-five minutes before my butt would become numb, and then the entire lower half of my body would fall asleep. Phone reservationists should not have numb butts because a numb butt does not a cheery phone reservationist make, and toward the end of every shift when I was supposed to be answering questions with quiet concern and authority, I found myself yelling NO YOU CANNOT RIDE IN THE CARGO BAY WITH YOUR CAT, ARE YOU INSANE?

Behold, there I was doing a job that stupid people before me had been able to do. And yes, I did consider parenthood a job. It was the most difficult job I'd ever had, a job where my boss called at least twice during the middle of the night, a job where my boss had to approve my bathroom breaks, a job that required me to wipe my boss's ass. And not only was I really good at it, but I was also stupid enough to love it.

After two months of sleepless nights we decided to try putting Leta to sleep in her crib and leaving her there for the duration of the evening. This experiment produced mixed results as some nights I was walking to her bedroom over twenty times to soothe her back to sleep or to plop that goddamn binky back in her face. Some of my friends thought I was insane and that I needed to let her cry it out right that instant be-cause it worked for them! And I totally gave them a cookie and encour-aged them to run for president.

I wasn't morally opposed to letting her cry it out; it's just that I didn't think she was ready for it. I wasn't ready for it. By the way her sleep habits were playing out I knew that I'd eventually have to give her a crash course in sleeping through the night, and I was certain it would be the hardest thing I would ever do in my life. It was hard enough to put her back in her crib when we made the decision that I shouldn't bring her back to bed with me after her first nightly feeding. That was my favorite part of the day, getting back into bed with her under my left arm, her soft furry hair brushing my chin, the smell of her head lulling me to sleep. It was beautiful and natural and magical, but then she started grunting and shooting firecrackers out of her ass. Sleeping directly next to the loudest baby on the planet proved nearly impossible.

So I started putting her back into her crib after the first feeding, and the first time I did it I cried all the way back to my bed, like I had just sent her off to college and she wasn't answering my calls. But that was the first time Jon was able to sleep over five hours in a row, and once we made that decision he consistently collected multiple hours of sleep, and that meant he was well rested enough that he could change more diapers and rub my feet and make me Pop-Tarts. I was still sleeping only two hours here and there because I was the feeder and official binky-putter-back-inner, but I had Pop-Tarts and rubbed feet and the world was once again okay.

But every night the trip to and from her room became more perilous as every single floorboard in our house creaked, and I swear they didn't creak before Leta was born. After she came to live with us they started to creak under the weight of our shadows. And they didn't creak softly or longingly. They creaked violently and adamantly, like an angry symphony of floorboards trying furiously to re-create the sounds of souls damned to hell, souls crying out for mercy. Even the thirty-five-pound dog caused the floors to creak.

Once Leta woke up, whether it was in the morning or from one of her naps, I set my watch and made sure that I got her back to sleep before the two-hour mark. She couldn't physically handle being awake for longer than that period of time and if we ignored that standard the PARTY WAS TOTALLY OVER. If we kept her awake even one minute over that two-hour mark, neither Jon nor I could console the beast that raged out of her screaming, violent limbs, and the switchover from beauty to beast was almost instantaneous.

These maddening sleep habits were one of many concerns we raised when we took her to her two-month checkup and torture session where she was weighed, measured, and injected with three potentially deadly diseases. Turns out she hadn't inherited her mother's aversion to needles, and she cried for all of four seconds after the final shot. I, however, saw the nurse make a movement toward my baby's leg and then vomited twice in the corner of the room.

She was twelve whole pounds—almost a baker's dozen!—and stretched out to twenty-four inches. I liked to tell people that she was two feet tall. The circumference of her head measured in the ninety-fifth percentile, meaning her head was bigger than the heads of 95 percent of all other babies her age. Oddly, this made me very proud. It was as if her brain was so big that it required extra storage space.

Her doctor gave us some upsetting news, however, when he diagnosed her with what is called torticollis plagiocephaly, a deformity in the shape of the head caused by favoring one side over the other. I'd noticed with some concern that when Leta was awake her head was positioned so that she was looking toward her right shoulder, and this caused the back of her head to grow into a diagonal slope. Her doctor was worried that the deformity had become so pronounced in just two months, so we made an appointment with a physical therapist in the following weeks to make sure that her neck muscles were developing correctly on both sides.

If you want to know how to scare the living shit out of a new mother, just utter the phrase TORTICOLLIS PLAGIOCEPHALY, and then hand her a prescription pad with the number of a SPECIALIST written on it, someone who is better trained with "these things." The condition was in no way life threatening, but I was a new mother and there was little difference to me between *mildly concerning* and *will totally kill your baby.*

Jon accepted the diagnosis in stride, but then again, he was preoccupied with thoughts of work and projects. I was almost jealous that he got to flee the physical confines of parenthood every day and focus on something completely unrelated to the survival of an infant. Although I knew he used his work as a distraction from the unpleasantness of what was going on at home, from the lingering image of his daughter's diagonal skull. My reaction to things was to cry. His was to flee.

That night we slept with Leta nestled between us. She was whimpering and aching from a 101 degree fever (a side effect of her immunizations), and I rested my hand on her belly all night long to feel the rise and fall of her breathing. I had never been so sad and worried and hopelessly wrapped up in another creature. I wanted to apologize to her all night, through her sobs and wails and half attempts at eating, for bringing her into this insane world where there are dangerous illnesses that she has to be protected against.

I was sorry about the shots. I was sorry that the shape of her head was distorted. I was sorry that the peanut butter and jelly sandwich I had the other day had given her bad gas. I was sorry that the dog loved to sniff her face and that his nose was really cold. I was sorry for dressing her in that onesie that was too small but was still so cute that I wanted her to wear it at least one more time. I was sorry that we had to pull her nightgown over her head, night after night after night. I was sorry that one day she'd have to figure out how to pay her own taxes and that we wouldn't pay them for her.

I was sorry that one day she would be old enough that when she was sick and had a fever I wouldn't be able to hold her and whisper her to sleep. I was sorry that I didn't ever want that day to come.

Most of my freelance web design work that used to bring in income during my pregnancy had dwindled to a very slow trickle. That was intentional, something I had planned because I knew I'd have a hard time juggling a baby and work. But there was one project that didn't want to end, there always is, so I enlisted my mother to watch the baby and the dog one afternoon so that I could tie up all the loose ends. I also used that opportunity to get out of the house for a few hours, so I drove the kids to my mother's house, better known as the International House of Treats. My mother was incapable of spending time with the baby or the dog without lavishing them with gifts, so whenever we saw my mother I could safely assume that her local Wal-Mart had recently been emptied of all pink pajamas and packaged sausages.

In addition to watching the baby while I grunted through some terrible design templates, my mother spent her day sneaking the dog large chunks of cheese under the counter. I didn't mind her giving the dog treats, and cheese happened to be his favorite, but my family never does anything in small quantities. We're big people with big appetites and big hands and big feet and we buy everything in bulk, and by the

end of the day my mother had given the dog enough cheese to consti-
pate an entire herd of bison. The truck smelled of dog cheese farts for a
week.

During the first few weeks of having a new baby I really enjoyed the
very rare instances that I could spend entire days away from the house
because it gave me a break in a frustrating routine consisting only of
feeding, catnapping, and changing a never-ending string of diapers.
Once I finally had the baby on a more predictable schedule it was hard
to spend the day away from the smells and textures and noise levels she
had become accustomed to, especially when spending the day away
involved my relatives, The Loudest People On Earth.

For instance, my stepfather would answer the telephone as if he were
trying to communicate from his living room with a deaf person locked
in a fallout shelter on the moon. I wanted to tell him, hey, I don't think
that deaf person can hear you, maybe if you SCREAMED A LITTLE
LOUDER THE WINDOWS WOULD EXPLODE AND THERE
WOULD BE ONE LESS BARRIER. My mother talked the exact same
way on the phone, as if she didn't trust technology and couldn't fathom
that someone five hundred miles away could hear her unless she was
S.H.R.I.E.K.I.N.G.

And then there was Granny, my eighty-year-old grandmother who
could not hear anything and so performed everything so forcibly that
even if she couldn't hear she would at least be able to feel the vibrations.
No one had ever opened a door so loudly, a door with no noticeable
creaking, a door with no obvious reason to be loud. She could make
that door loud, just like she could clomp around the house in slippers
causing the foundation of the house to tremble. HOW CAN YOU
POSSIBLY CLOMP IN HOUSE SLIPPERS? And NO, you are not

allowed to go wake up "that baby" to squeeze her face, you insane slipper-clomping door opener!

By the time we headed home after a day with my family I was a ball of nerves, having dodged catastrophe after catastrophe with the loud phone talkers. Leta somehow managed to sleep through four openings and closings of the garage door from hell, a conference call involving my mother and the speaker phone, and my stepfather's encounter with a package of deli meat that would not open. I had never been so mad at a slice of turkey in my life.

When I was a child I knew the proper terms for the sexual anatomies of both girls and boys and wasn't afraid to remind my grandmother to wash my vagina when giving me a bath. My grandmother, however, couldn't believe she had raised a son who could in good conscience teach his own kids to use such foul language. Oh the horror of her grandchild uttering PENIS! You might as well arm your kids with a gun and teach them how to shoplift! Penis is of course the gateway drug to felony misdemeanor.

At the age of four I was also under the impression that the penis was also called a delicate. The only way I could get my then seven-year-old brother to stop tickling me was to kick him in the delicate. It worked every time! My father had to pull me aside and tell me that boys had delicate parts and that I could permanently injure my brother's delicate if I kept kicking him there. Years later when I was able to spell I noticed that the washing machine had a delicate cycle, and I could not for the life of me figure out how boys could detach their penises to wash them in the washing machine. And where was the vagina cycle? I wanted to detach my vagina and stick it in the washing machine. That only seemed fair.

Jon's mother had also taught him the proper terms for his anatomy, but when she taught him that a vagina was a vagina he thought she said China. For years he would silently gasp when anyone referred to the country or to the tableware, and once when he was at his friend's house and his friend's mother began singing "China Girl" he could not believe this woman was openly talking about her China. HAD SHE NO DECENCY?

But Jon and I struggled with what we were going to call Leta's anatomy when she was old enough to start talking about it. I did want her to know that she had a vagina, and we would teach her all the medical terms pertaining to her AREA, but when we talked about it casually, I thought that calling it a vagina would get tiring. Vagina is such a laborious word. It's got three distinct syllables and you almost have to chew the word to get it out. What we were looking for was something cuter. Vagina was not cute.

We also had to consider the fact that whatever we taught her to call it would have its meaning completely altered in her mind. If we taught her to call it her PARTS then whenever she heard the word PART she'd either be mortified or chuckle wickedly. And then there was that one time the ultrasound technician called it a CHEESEBURGER, but I didn't want her to have to think about her vagina every time she pulled up to a drive-thru.

Some terms we considered:

Bug

There

That Place

Um, you know (and then pointing in the general direction)

Certain Things Unspoken

Bottom System

When some of my more conservative friends found out that we were even considering assigning a nickname to Leta's private parts they freaked out. Didn't I know that encouraging such aberrant behavior meant that she'd grow up and nickname the severed limbs in her deep freezer? And I assured them, look, it's not like we were going to call it her Wallace or her Supreme Chancellor Palpatine. GIVE ME SOME CREDIT.

In the end we decided on BUNKY because it was cute, and there was no possibility of it being confused with any other inanimate object. Except that I guess one of my friends knows this guy whose grand-mother's name is Bunky. WHAT ARE THE CHANCES OF THAT? And why did she have to tell me because now when I hear the word all I can think of is an imaginary silver-haired woman wearing a floral apron and garden clogs. That image lodged itself into my brain and now whenever I talk about my bunky I can't help but envision a vagina preparing a pot roast and then sewing the button back on a festive Christmas sweater.

Dear Leta,

Today you are officially eight weeks old. I am sitting here typ-ing this as you lie sleeping next to me. Over the weekend your father and I discovered that if we place you on your stomach you will actually sleep longer than five minutes at a time. This morning, in fact, I had to wake you up after three whole hours of sleeping soundly on your stomach, and when I rolled you over you had the cutest case of Binky Face, all mushed and covered in binky-shaped indentations.

I wish they made Binky Face bread tins so that I could bake a loaf of banana bread in the shape of your sleeping profile, and then instead of trying to eat your chubby cheeks I could just eat the banana bread. That would probably be better for both of us.

Yesterday I read in one of the dozens of medical books we bought since your birth that babies your age can sometimes wrap their fingers around objects that are held close to their hands. So we decided to test that theory out, and when we held a small rattle close to your right hand you reached out and wrapped your fingers around that thing so hard that it almost snapped in two. And then, proving once again that you probably have ancestors from the planet Krypton, you began waving that rattle around like you were flagging down a plane.

Your father and I got so excited that we almost had to change each other's diapers, and we sat there cheering, "GO BABY GO!" At that moment I totally forgave you for the hours and hours—and did I mention hours?—of sleep I have lost getting out of bed at night to walk into your room to put the binky back in your mouth.

Sometimes you snort loudly in your sleep. Gigantic snorts that remarkably never wake you up. For the past couple of weeks when you have been attempting to sleep on your back, you have been waking yourself up by smacking yourself in the face repeatedly. I did a Google search on this flailing arm phenomenon (other recent Google searches include: "baby poop looks like caramel" and "healthy baby poop" and "infant hair loss Rogaine") and I couldn't find any professional advice on how to restrain your arms so that you can get some sleep. There have been nights when I've brought you back to bed with me that you have punched me in the nose with your little clenched fist and I've had to walk around the next day with a swollen nostril.

We've tried swaddling you, and in the first month of your life swaddling totally worked and you looked like a little frog-caterpillar hybrid. But your arms have become strong enough in the past month that you can break free of any of our swaddles, your father's swaddles included, and your father could swaddle a full-grown octopus and it wouldn't be able to wiggle its arms.

A side effect of your Flailing Infant Arm Syndrome is your discovery of your right hand, which you like to chew on at every possible opportunity. Aside from being very cute and very loud—the air you suck around your fist tends to slurp and often it sounds like a four-hundred-pound man passing garlic farts—your hand-chewing is also very drooly, dripping with drool, and if I don't keep up with the drool the entire right side of your face becomes slimy with drool bubbles. You don't seem to mind at all, but of course, you don't mind sticking your sock-covered foot into your seedy caramel poop as I change your diaper, thus forcing me to do YET ANOTHER load of laundry. I can't wait to teach you how to do laundry. I could use the help.

I look forward to this next month with you, to more coos and noises and near giggles, to more of the moments like the other night when I was feeding you at 1:30 AM and you kicked your sleeping father in the head. Your father and I love you more than you could possibly know, and you won't know or understand just how much until you have a child of your own. Just please don't have that child when you're still a teenager. Which reminds me: you're not allowed to date until you are twenty-five.

Love, Mama

CHAPTER NINE

The Dive That Turned Into a Belly Flop

*B*efore Leta was born Jon and I talked at length about what we would do if I slipped into a postpartum funk, but for some reason I didn't think it would ever happen, especially since I had made it through those first crucial months. But the funk finally happened, and it wasn't so much a simple slipping into as it was a full-fledged belly flop.

For several weeks I felt like I was fighting a losing battle. I was doing everything I knew how to do to cope with feelings of hopelessness and frustration and an overwhelming sense of failure. But the cumulative loss of sleep and genetic predisposition toward depression totally body slammed me, and I spent several days locked in the house crying and wanting to puke.

Jon spent several days at work picking up his phone only to have me hang up on him. At night I would beg him to stay home the next day, and he would often say that while work was no fun it was far better than the sound of my screaming, not to mention the endless squawking coming from the nursery. And then every day he'd go to work to escape us.

I experienced a few days of intense postpartum blues during the first two weeks of Leta's life, but they subsided, the weather got better, my body healed, and soon I found myself getting out of the house and putting makeup on every day. The sleep deprivation was hard, but everything else was manageable because Leta seemed to be a relatively easy baby.

Almost everything I'd read said that a baby's fussiness peaked at about six weeks of age, and when Leta turned six weeks I almost threw a celebration because I thought I might be out of the woods. But Leta became fussy at six weeks, and her fussiness only increased with each passing day. I don't know if her temperament changed, I got worn down, or the lethal combination of both, but she rejected all my attempts to establish a schedule, and I spent days on end trying to soothe her incessant screaming. She screamed for hours every day. By the end of the day she was so tired from not sleeping that she was too frustrated to eat. Then she became too hungry to sleep and would lie there screaming. My daily life felt like torture. I struggled to make it from hour to hour. I felt like I didn't know what I was doing. I was trying to find the humor in all of it, but I couldn't ignore the crushing misery any longer.

There were many things about parenthood that I understood intellectually. I knew that this period of her life was only temporary and that things would eventually get better. I knew that I was a good mother and that I was meeting her needs as a baby. But depression isn't about understanding things intellectually. It's about an overshadowing emotional spiral that makes coping with anything nearly impossible.

I just couldn't cope with the screaming. I couldn't cope with her not eating. I couldn't cope with the constant pacing and rocking back and forth to make sure she didn't start crying. I was sick with anxiety. I wanted to throw up all day long. There were moments during her screaming when I had to set her down and walk away and regain perspective on life, because in those very dark moments of screaming I felt like I had destroyed mine.

The anxiety robbed me of all sleep. Every day as the morning turned into afternoon I started to get sick at my stomach with the prospect of what the evening brought: screaming and feeling totally helpless, my boobs filling up with milk that she wouldn't eat.

Most of the literature I'd read about depression medication and breastfeeding indicated that the benefits of breastfeeding far outweighed the possibility of the baby receiving small amounts of the medication through the breast milk. I also thought that it was more important that my daughter have a mother who could cope—a mother who wasn't sobbing uncontrollably during diaper changes—than it was for her to have a mother who was too proud to admit defeat.

I was throwing up my hands. I couldn't do this unmedicated, and it was a decision I did not make lightly. I'd read everything I could get my hands on concerning postpartum depression in the mother and how it affected the development of the baby. I'd talked with my doctor and friends who had experienced the same debilitating feelings. Going off depression medication before my pregnancy was so awful that I didn't ever want to have to face that nightmare again. And for weeks I had been silently whispering to myself, *Fight this! Fight this!* But I lost the fight, and I was really scared.

I was scared that the meds might not work. I was scared that the side effect of fatigue combined with my already near deadly sleep deprivation would render me as useless as I was off the meds. I was scared of what it all meant, about me, about who I thought I was.

But I felt like I didn't have a choice, the hopelessness was just too overwhelming. I wanted to look back on that time fondly and remember her smiles, not her screaming. And too often I didn't even notice when she was smiling.

During my pregnancy I saw signs that I was turning into my mother when instead of using free time to sleep I spent it folding socks and washing the bathroom mirror. But I thought that I was just experiencing a nesting instinct and that I would go back to my usual low-energy self once the baby was here.

The baby's birth, however, seemed to have tripped a latent portion of my DNA that caused at least half of my brain to be consumed at all times with the thought of chores that needed to be done. In the time it took Jon to change Leta's morning diaper I could have the dishwasher unloaded, bagels toasted, coffee brewed, bed made, and dog pooped, and that was only if the diaper hadn't leaked. On the frequent occasion that she was covered in pee and Jon had to take a few extra minutes to change her clothes, I could wallpaper the living room and mow the lawn.

When I was a kid I hated this about my mother, her constant need to get something done around the house. If she was talking to a friend on the phone she was also dusting the living room or hauling dirty clothes to the washing machine. On Saturday mornings she was up at the crack of dawn vacuuming her bedroom or scrubbing the tiles in the shower, and I remember thinking, *doesn't she know the Smurfs are on?* How could she mop the kitchen floor when Gargamel was chasing Smurfette with a stick?

Once I became a mother I realized that free time was one of the many luxuries people give up when they decide to procreate. I kind of understood this going into parenthood, but it's not something you can TRULY appreciate, like everything else about parenthood, until it drops on your head like a piano shoved out of a window eighty stories high.

Free time was the four minutes it took Jon to change Leta's diaper; it was the one minute I had to use the bathroom after I set her down in the crib; it was the thirty seconds she would remain calm in the car seat after we returned from the grocery store. On the infrequent occasion that she remained napping for longer than twenty minutes I felt like a teenage boy who had just locked himself in the bathroom with a stack of porn magazines, like OH MY GOD, THE POSSIBILITIES. WHERE DO I EVEN BEGIN?

Before Leta was born I used to hate to run errands, and I would put off going to the grocery store until the milk was so expired that it had grown arms, legs, and a fully functioning liver. But all that changed, and I wanted to go to the grocery store every day if only to see other human beings who spoke in sentences and could wipe their own asses. It reassured me that there was living, breathing life outside of the twilight zone existence of taking care of a creature whose primary means of communication was through her bowels.

One night Jon let me go to the grocery store alone, something a new father should be very wary of letting a new mother do, because once I was behind that steering wheel I became drunk with the freedom. I honestly thought that the car might sprout wings and take off in the air, and I was flooded with grand ideas of escaping to Montana where I could assume a new identity and drink martinis and sleep in until 8 AM.

It would have been so easy to have kept driving, forever. Maybe no one would notice I was gone!

But five minutes into shopping at the grocery store I started to miss that little screaming baby at home. WHY WAS I MISSING HER? That was MY time. Why was I thinking about her little cold feet and her fuzzy hair and the yummy creases in her baby thighs? WHY WHY WHY?

So I didn't gas up and drive to Montana, but instead came back home and immediately went into the house to smell the back of her neck. And while she was still under Jon's watchful eye I landscaped the backyard and remodeled the basement.

Desperate times call for desperate measures, and after several days of Leta's unwillingness to eat a full meal during the day I found myself on the phone with La Leche League, otherwise known in this household as The Boob Nazis. I was worried about my milk supply, that somehow my boobs might dry up because Leta would rather stare at a blank wall than eat, and I needed some professional advice.

Nikki, the La Leche League leader in my area, assured me that my milk supply would be fine, as long as Leta was eating at some point during the day, and the only thing I should worry about was becoming engorged because then my boobs would tell my body to stop producing so much milk. I asked her if I should just pump if I became engorged, and she answered in all seriousness, "Why, certainly, go ahead and pump, and store away that milk in the freezer so that in three years when you decide to give up breastfeeding, you'll have some extra you can give your baby."

Blink.

Blink, blink.

Three years?

Blink.

Three as in the one that comes after two?

My baby would be walking and talking in three years, and walking and talking might not be the perfect ingredients for a comfortable breastfeeding relationship, at least not for me and my boobs who didn't want to be walked up to. Many kudos to the woman who could continue breastfeeding her child through toddlerhood, but in my household there was only one person who was allowed to have a nickname for my chest and that person finished teething over thirty-eight years ago.

During Leta's first physical therapy session we got a better diagnosis for her head and neck condition and were instructed to give her a lot of tummy time where she'd lie on her stomach and lift up her head to strengthen her abdominal muscles. Leta, unfortunately, had been cursed with two parents who suffer varying degrees of obsessive-compulsive disorder, and she spent two weeks of her life on her stomach, her mother and father cheering maniacally from the sidelines. That exercise was a mixed blessing, however, because not only did she now know how to hold up her head, but she also knew how to HOLD UP HER HEAD, DEAR GOD.

Apparently, there is nothing more exciting or fulfilling in this world than to hold up one's head, and why eat or sleep when you could hold up your head? When I tried to feed her during the day she'd stop after maybe a minute and then look at me like, *WAIT! You tricked me! A minute ago I was holding up my head and now I'm not holding up my head and I need to hold up my head!* And then she'd root and contort her body in an attempt to get into a position where she could hold up her head. And her thundering sigh of relief could be heard in Minnesota.

The good news was that Leta wouldn't have to wear a helmet. We'd been so overzealous with her neck exercises that the therapist projected that the shape of her head would resolve itself within two months. Hoorah for OCD! The bad news was that in the next month or two she'd be learning how to reach for things and how to sit up on her own, and OH MY GOD, she'd never eat or sleep again because she'd be reaching and sitting and holding up her head. I had a decision to make, did I want my child to develop normally, or did I want to sleep? AND I WAS HAVING A HARD TIME CHOOSING.

One Saturday afternoon my mother agreed to take Leta for a few hours so that Jon and I could go see a movie. A movie in a movie theater. A whole movie with opening credits and a plot and closing credits with actors and music and a life lesson and everything. A MOVIE!

Jon and I hadn't seen a movie since Leta was born, not in a movie theater or even in our own home, as that would have required a huge chunk of undivided attention. I hadn't been willing to make a commitment to a one hour and forty-eight minute story line, not when there were four loads of laundry to do and the bathroom sink needed to be scrubbed.

Plus, it was almost impossible to time any sort of outing with Leta's feedings, especially since her relationship with the bottle was sort of sketchy. Sometimes she'd drink from one, but usually she'd scream as if it were trying to drink her.

We decided that we wanted to see something memorable and worthy of the effort of arranging an outing, because OH MY GOD THE

ARRANGING, so we chose to see a movie based on a book. Timing everything so that we could make that movie on time was like planning a wedding, and in case you don't remember, my husband and I eloped because I didn't ever want to have to plan a wedding. YUCK.

We had to get ourselves showered, the baby dressed, the bags packed, the milk pumped, the bottles ready, the car seat base ready to switch cars, and then I had to feed the baby while my mother and stepfather waited in the living room. And I really, really hated it when people were waiting on me while I breastfed—I'd get performance anxiety and start to worry that maybe right then, RIGHT THAT SECOND, my boobs were going to dry up and everyone's day would be ruined! Ruined because of my boobs!

With twenty minutes until show time, Jon and I kissed Leta goodbye (and there were four whole seconds there when I honestly thought of backing out of the whole arrangement, the thought of being away from Leta for four whole hours made my soul shrivel up), climbed into the car, and headed downtown. We rolled down the windows, opened the sunroof, and turned the stereo so loud that we couldn't hear each other screaming WE ARE GOING TO SEE A MOVIE, AMERICA!

I had never been so excited to see a movie in my entire life. I had probably never been so excited about a car ride in my entire life, a car ride with no car seat and no screaming. Well, there was screaming, but it was celebratory screaming, not the type of screaming that can't be consoled with rocking or walking around or turning on the hair dryer or PUTTING THE BABY ON THE WASHING MACHINE AND SHE STILL WON'T STOP SCREAMING.

We were screaming and singing, and the wind was flowing through our hair, and we were going to see a movie. (A MOVIE!) Maybe life was looking up. Maybe we were going to come out the other end of the dark cave that had become our home, and life was going to be really, really good. Maybe.

But four blocks from the movie theater we ran into a police barricade. And they wouldn't let people through. So Jon turned the car around to head up a different street, another street just FOUR BLOCKS AWAY FROM THE MOVIE THEATER, and that street was blocked, too. So he turned again, and we couldn't get past another police barricade because that day, that one right there, THE DAY WE ARRANGED TO GO SEE A MOVIE, THE DAY I HAD TO BREASTFEED WHILE MY MOTHER AND STEPFATHER WAITED IN THE OTHER ROOM, that day was the Salt Lake Marathon.

And we couldn't get past that barricade.

And we were stuck in traffic.

On our movie day.

And we couldn't go forward and we couldn't back up and my soul shriveled up into black nothingness and was wearing black tights and black mascara and started listening to The Cure.

We spent the next forty-five minutes IN OUR CAR, four blocks away from the movie theater. Every fifteen minutes or so Jon would turn and ask me, "I shouldn't talk to you right now, huh?"

I'd never been so devastated.

When we finally got to the movie theater the only movie we could still see in time was a romantic comedy, and it was terrible and awful and made me cringe in so many places, but it was the best movie I had ever seen.

Dear Leta,

I have fed you twice a night every night for the past eighty-four days, and I have to ask you: aren't you full yet?

This week you turn three months old, and your father and I can't believe we have made it this far. The past few weeks have seemed like some sort of hazy acid trip, not that we would know what an acid trip feels like because we would never drop acid, no not ever. Drugs are bad and you should say no to drugs, but Advil is totally okay, and can I tell you how happy I am that I get to take Advil again? When I was pregnant with you I wasn't allowed to take Advil, and whenever I had a headache or a sore muscle your father would take a handful of Advil and stand close to me in hopes that his nearness would soothe me. Now I just sprinkle a few capsules in my breakfast in the morning.

Things have been hazy because we're still trying to figure out your sleep schedule. We've made huge progress since last month, at least in terms of night sleeping, but the day sleeping thing is causing your chemically imbalanced mother to hide in the closet and scratch sores that don't exist.

We put you to bed every night sometime between 6 PM and 8 PM depending on how you've slept during the day, and we always go through the same ritual of bathing you, dressing you, and feeding you. This ritual is our favorite part of the day, and one night last week your father was late coming home from work and I had to bathe you by myself. I have never seen your father so devastated! He missed bathtime with his little

Thumper, a nickname we've given you because whenever we lie you down on the changing table you immediately begin thumping it with both of your legs so violently that the whole changing table shakes.

You LOVE the changing table. You love it more than the swing or the bouncy seat, and sometimes you love it more than being held by me or your father and we promise not to hold that against you, at least not until you come home with piercings in your face and then I WILL TOTALLY HOLD IT AGAINST YOU.

During the night you will usually sleep in stretches that last anywhere from three to five hours, and you will also go right back to sleep after you eat. When you wake up in the morning at about 7 AM you are always smiling, and Leta, those morning smiles are the reason your father and I decided to have kids. Your smile is brighter than the sun, the most beautiful addition to my life, and I would forsake all the Advil in the world to see it every morning.

And then there is the day-sleeping, or more accurately, the complete absence of day-sleeping, and when you don't sleep during the day you are the crankiest baby on the planet. So cranky, in fact, that sometimes you scream. Can we please talk about the screaming? Is the screaming really necessary?

I have received a lot of advice concerning your screaming, people who think you might have reflux or an ear infection, people who think I need to stop breastfeeding you, people who think I need to start feeding you Cheerios already. And I think this may be the first instance where I take a stand as your mother, the one person who knows you best, and declare that the only reason you are screaming is because you are tired. Your little body needs rest, and when you take naps during the day you are glorious, the most precious and wonderful and awesome baby that ever came out of a womb. When you don't take naps you are *HORRIFYING* and there isn't a window in the world that I wouldn't throw you out of.

For the past five days you have slept well both at night and during the day and you have only screamed *ONCE*, and that was yesterday when I tried to put you in the BabyBjörn, the contraption that holds you to my chest so that I can walk with my hands free. I couldn't figure out how the straps worked, and you were being very patient, and then somehow I flipped you upside-down and the strap wrapped itself around your face, and I would scream, too, if my mother mushed my nose between two metal snaps.

We love you, little Thumper.

Love, Mama

CHAPTER TEN

Your Biological Clock Is a Dumbass

One of the saddest endeavors I'd ever been a part of was packing all of Leta's 0–3 month clothing into labeled boxes and storing them away in the basement where they'd remain until we had another baby—HA! ANOTHER BABY? The logistics of more than one TOTALLY BOGGLED MY MIND. Leta would never be able to wear those clothes again, and as I folded each nightgown into a box my heart broke just thinking about how much money her father and I would be spending on clothes in the next eighteen years. And I suddenly realized, HOLY HELL, this baby will one day turn into a teenager, and why didn't anyone tell me?

Why couldn't we have her go from toddlerhood straight to self-sufficiency and bypass all the bad hair and braces and lessons in menstruation and endless nights of crying because her boobs aren't big enough?

And what if she wanted to have her own blog? I HADN'T THOUGHT ABOUT THAT. Dear God, the Internet wouldn't be big enough to hold all her complaining, and I could totally see her getting kicked out of school because she'd written stories about her teachers, and what would I say? I would say *If you're going to write stories about your teachers at least make them unrecognizable, for crying out loud!* And then we'd go shopping for a padded bra.

What would happen when she found out that I once talked about throwing her out the window? I WAS KIDDING, LETA! I wouldn't really throw you out the window! I might pull your toes until you scream, but the window thing . . . a JOKE! And that time I called you a frog, I meant that lovingly. Frogs are great! I love frogs!

Now that she was wearing clothing from Big & Tall I didn't dress her in as many frilly outfits as I had when she was smaller. She was more mature than that now, and so I dressed her in long pants and sophisticated onesies, all without lace and bows. We are not bow people, we Armstrongs, and never would anyone be able to convince me that it was perfectly okay to put a bow in her nonexistent hair. Really, is there anything more frightening than a bow on a bald head? WHAT IS IT DOING THERE except making a baby look like a PIN CUSHION?

Jon did make me promise, however, that I would never take Leta out in public with bare feet because apparently nothing screams NE-GLECT! like a sockless baby. It's not that I was struggling with deep and unresolved sock issues, I just didn't see why she always had to wear socks when she wasn't even using her feet. But then, I was also the type of mother who would rather put tin foil in the windows to keep out the light than buy a proper set of blinds, and OH MY GOD what my kid is going to say about me on her website.

Some days were really good.

Some days started with bacon and biscuits and then more bacon because the first round of bacon wasn't enough. Some days had foot rubs and flowers and an extra thirty minutes of sleep, delicious and indulgent. Some days the drugs seemed to work and I felt like I was born to do this, and when I looked at her and I didn't remember the stretch marks or the constipation or the episiotomy or the bladder infections or the constantly malfunctioning left boob that woke me up every four days with a clogged milk duct or the hemorrhoids or the bloating or the nausea or the tremendous weight gain.

Some days I enjoyed living in the moment and treasured her little feet and fingers and squeals and excessive drool, because I knew she would never be this little again. Some days I hoped she never grew up.

But most days were really, really bad.

Some days she started screaming only a half hour after she woke up, and I immediately wanted to hit the reset button. Some days the drugs didn't work, and the isolation of spending my entire day with someone who couldn't tell me what she wanted, PLEASE JUST TELL ME WHAT YOU WANT, spread like a disease in my body, choking me and rendering me paralyzed.

Some days I remembered the ongoing physical pain of bringing and having this child in the world, and I wondered how much more my body could take. Some days I made it to 11 AM, and then I made it to 2 PM, and then I'd try, try, try to make it until Jon came home, and when I did I felt simultaneously triumphant and beaten down.

Some days I stared eternity in the face and thought about how many diapers I would change that would only get dirty again, towels I would wash that would only become soiled, dishes I would load into the dishwasher that we'd use to eat on again and again, and I felt useless, as if I was fighting a battle that couldn't be won.

Some days my life was reduced to an hour by hour game of survival and I didn't feel like I'd make it another fifteen minutes, and I couldn't stop crying.

A friend once asked me whether or not I liked my job, and at the time I was working full-time at a web design shop in Los Angeles. My answer was that I loved my job approximately three days out of every month, and during the other twenty-seven or so days our relationship was more platonic, at times resembling the rocky relationship of two college roommates who happen to be on their periods at the same time.

I figured that three whole days' worth of love was much more than most people could claim about their employment, and so I didn't mind lugging my hungover body into the office most of the week to deal with Account People Who Wear Panty Hose Even Though No Dress Code Requires Them To Do So. For three days every month I got to work on an original design, and then I would spend the next four weeks redesigning and tearing apart that design, all to the specifications of those Account People and clients who thought that the Internet was a person who lived inside their computers.

I actually worked for a client once who asked me to program their homepage so that when a user brought it up on a browser it would disable the printing function on their computer. They didn't want anyone printing out their website because they were worried that someone would steal their great ideas, the great ideas that they were *putting on the Internet* for thousands of people to read. I asked them if they also wanted me to include a piece of code that would break a user's fingers, thus preventing anyone from printing or even writing down their great ideas, and they asked me if they could get in trouble for that. Sometimes parenthood doesn't seem so bad.

Some of my friends at the time said that they were envious of my job, that I got to work with big-name clients and that I got to play on the Internet all day long, and from the perspective of someone who was washing dishes and waiting tables for hours on end, I can see how my job would have seemed alluring. But the reality was much less glamorous than the idea of it, because there's nothing fancy or prestigious about spending forty hours on one background color because someone in charge can't decide if he likes purple or *dark* purple.

Maybe all jobs are like this in the sense that there are the good parts and the bad parts, the bad parts occupying the majority of the space because it is a JOB after all. If you have a job where there are more good parts than bad parts then you've obviously made a deal with the Devil and you're going to spend the rest of eternity being tortured by fork-wielding elves to make up for the imbalance. I'm just saying.

I remember when I was single and living alone and wondering what it would be like to be married and have a family, and whenever I saw people with kids at the park I couldn't wait to have my own kids to play with at the park, because that's what having a family was going to be like. Playing at the park. Having a family was going to be so fun, and there would be ice cream cones and tricycles and round baby cheeks and everyone would be smiling all the time. I couldn't wait to have a kid that I could dress in a soccer uniform, someone whose hair I could braid, someone I could train to say mean things to the Mormons.

And I know that what I'm about to say is completely obvious, and it will be the least profound thing I have ever written. But to those who have suffered the unmerciful pangs of an angry biological clock, who have felt weak in the knees at the sight of a newborn baby, who daydream like I did about what your own kids will look like, what the biological clock isn't telling you is that the job of motherhood is nothing like what you think it will be.

Yes, there were baby smiles and giggles, although Leta only giggled for her father. Or when I had just left the room. She was evil that way.

There were transcendental moments when I'd look at her and she'd look at me and there were traces of recognition and THE WORLD STOOD STILL I LOVED HER SO MUCH.

But there was all this other stuff that I hadn't bargained for, and I felt foolish for being so unprepared. The day to day minutiae of raising a baby was at times so boring that I wanted to bang my head against the changing table. There were only so many ways to entertain a three-month-old baby (Let's walk into the kitchen again! Let's look out the window! Here, chew on my finger!), and I knew it would only get worse from there. In the next year I'd be repeating words all day long, reading the same books over and over and over again, and changing diapers that would redefine my entire definition of offensive.

I was discovering that motherhood was just like any other job, that the good and fun parts were there, it just wasn't good and fun all the time or even most of the time. I now understood that the family with the kids at the park had to get those kids dressed and fed and into the car and that on the way to the park the kids probably all threw tantrums and spit at each other. And then they had to get back into the car, drive home while everyone was complaining about how hot it was, and then they had to feed them dinner, get them ready for bed, and fight them to brush their teeth. And those kids probably didn't even have the redeeming fresh baby smell that made so much of this job endurable.

· · ·

Books about early childhood development like to remind you to speak out loud to a baby all day long so that the little seedlings of language can take root in the mush of their brains. And when I say mush I mean it lovingly yet truthfully, because COME ON. I could have barked at Leta all day long and she would have found it just as instructional as if I were reading her a dictionary.

To prevent myself from absentmindedly going hours without saying anything, which happened many, many times—YOU try talking to a person who refuses to answer you or to give you any indication that she can differentiate your voice from the sound of the dishwasher—I developed the strategy of describing everything I did. This meant that I was talking all the time, nonstop, hours and hours without stopping:

"Right now I am lying you down on the bed, Leta. And while you lie there flailing your arms I am going to go turn on the television so that we can watch *Pyramid*, hosted by Donny Osmond who is a Mormon just like Grandmommy. *Pyramid* is our new favorite show, isn't it? It has nothing to do with Donny Osmond, who is very cute and all, and I know he sits at the right hand of God or whatever, but he has all the charisma of a lima bean. I'll never force you to eat lima beans, Leta, not like Grandmommy forced me. I'll also never force you to sing songs about how much you should want to grow up and become a missionary and thus a mindless cog in the wheel that is cultural imperialism. But I digress!

"We like *Pyramid* because it is fun to try and guess what these crazy people are trying to describe, isn't it? And when we do guess correctly we feel good about ourselves, because we're smart enough to know that when they say, 'Not winning, but . . . ' the correct answer is 'LOSING!' And when they say, 'Not a bride, but a . . . ' we say 'GROOM!' And the

thrill of it is exhilarating! Kind of what it feels like to drink a lot of coffee! And inevitably the word 'movie' will come up and the person describing the word will say, 'You go to the cinema to see a . . . ' and of
course the answer is 'MOVIE!' but the person who is supposed to guess
will invariably just sit there, dumb as a stick, and go, 'Huh? Guh?
Whah??' AS IF YOU WOULD EVER GO TO THE CINEMA TO
SEE ANYTHING BUT A MOVIE. THE WORLD IS A PIECE OF
CRAP."

That was the exact script of my day, really, just an incoherent string
of verbalizations that I hoped would stick in her mush. But I found that
I couldn't stop describing things even after we put her to bed, and by
the end of the night I'd given Jon a blow-by-blow commentary on how
I was brushing my teeth—"up and down and up and down, and now
the toothpaste is foaming, like an angry dog or maybe a washing machine that has been loaded with too much detergent, and now I'm spitting and isn't that gross." It got so out of hand that I fully expected Leta
to stop in the middle of one of her screaming fits and turn to me and
say, "WOULD YOU PLEASE JUST SHUT UP ALREADY."

Leta's screaming got really bad one week, not that I should have been
able to notice a difference in magnitude—is shrill any different from
really, really shrill? But one day her screams were shrill, and the next day
her screams were SO NOT KIDDING.

She'd been grabbing at both of her ears, so I decided to take her to
the doctor to find out if she was suffering from an ear infection. And I
won't lie, a baby with an ear infection was one of my worst nightmares,
right up there with being tickled to death or being force-fed black lico-

rice, The Worst Tasting Taste in All of Tasteland. But I was almost hoping that she had an ear infection because then they could give her an antibiotic, and then maybe the shrill screaming would come to an end. An ear infection would at least have been an explanation.

So I took her to the doctor and while we sat in the waiting room we watched other mothers chase after their shrieking, mobile toddlers and I caught a glimpse of what my life was going to be like in the next couple of years. It was like I was watching a videotape of my own execution, the volume deafeningly loud, and when one little boy threw himself on the floor and began pounding his arms and legs in a whirlwind thrashing of anger, all because his mom wouldn't let him tear the covers off of all the magazines—mean, unloving mother!—I felt the dull blade of the guillotine slice into my neck, my head tumbling off my body and into a jeering crowd of cannibalistic three-year-olds ready to gouge out my eyes and teeth with crayons.

Before the doctor checked her ears she stuck Leta on the scale and we were both startled at the number that popped up on the digital readout: 14 LBS, 8 OZ. My child had more than doubled her weight since we brought her home from the hospital. This made no sense because 1) Leta didn't really eat during the day, and 2) LETA DIDN'T EAT DURING THE DAY. I told the doctor that I'd been worried about her eating habits, and she looked at me like *ARE YOU KIDDING? YOU MEAN YOU AREN'T FEEDING HER BACON GREASE?* Which led me to believe that Jon was feeding her Twinkies behind my back.

The doctor then checked both of her ears for signs of infection, and not only did she not find any infection, she didn't even find any Twinkies. In fact, she found Leta to be the model of perfect health, a tragic diagnosis as that meant Leta was just irritable. There was no antibiotic for irritability. Ear infections would clear up in a matter of days, whereas irritability would last a lifetime, lifetime, lifetime. (Yes, that was an echo, symbolic of the vast canyon of misery ahead of me as mother of a screaming person who refused to stop screaming. And at the end of my life when Leta gave the eulogy at my funeral no one would understand a word of it because it will be ONE. LONG. STRING. OF. SCREAMS.)

When we bought the dishwasher during our kitchen remodel we also bought a garbage disposal as a new dishwasher won't work without one. And the dishwasher was our key to eternal salvation, remember? When we died we would go to heaven like all the other dishwasher-owning parents who sterilize bottles. Except, I was still a little confused as to how someone who bottle fed their baby could end up in heaven, even if they did sterilize the nipples, because God had himself decreed that mothers who don't breastfeed their babies go to hell, and by extension the non-breastfed baby is doomed to an eternity of shoveling coal alongside all the goblins of Hell. This was all discussed in the New Testament.

Against our better judgment we bought both items at a popular electronics store, also known as The Store for Masochists, but only because 1) the dishwasher was on sale and 2) this particular electronics store had special parking spaces for pregnant women. I was six months pregnant at the time, and the special parking space was like a corporate-sponsored invitation to eat whatever I wanted. No matter how big my ass became, no matter how wide the swipe of my waddle, those people had my back. I could swell to the size of a moose, and I wouldn't ever have to walk more than thirty feet from my car to buy a stereo. They really, really cared.

The disposal we bought came with a twelve-year manufacturer's warranty, which meant that it shouldn't have broken during THE NEXT TWELVE YEARS. Other than the seven dead bodies we shoved down the drain we hadn't used the disposal for anything more than to grind up a few leftover mushy peas, and they were mushy as mushy peas could sometimes be. But one weekend when the disposal still had eleven years and six months left on its warranty, it started leaking! Out the side! All over our new cabinetry! Onto our wood floors! And the usually serene and patient Husband, who normally stood by to watch the usually depraved and chemically imbalanced Wife lose her shit, TOTALLY LOST HIS SHIT.

So the family with no shit piled into the truck and headed to the electronics store, disassembled and leaking disposal in hand, to see if we could piece our shit together again. But this time we couldn't park in the special parking space because I was no longer pregnant (THANK THE LORD GOD JESUS!) and we had to park in the non-pregnant parking space and walk an extra twenty feet to the door. We found this inconvenience totally unacceptable as we were living in America and shouldn't have to walk an extra twenty feet for anything. AM I RIGHT? AM I RIGHT? This is the best country on Earth! WE DON'T WALK NOWHERE FOR NUTHING. Damn straight.

I carried the still-under-warranty disposal and Jon had Leta, the only member of this family with anything resembling pieced together shit, strapped to his chest in the BabyBjörn, her chubby, innocent cheeks facing outward, her arms and legs poking out the sides like a jumping jack frozen in midair. We marched right up to the Returns/Exchanges counter, plopped the leaking disposal on the counter and started re-counting our long-winded nightmare to the girl standing on the other side. Her eyes immediately glazed over. The girl had BRACES, for God's sake, CLEAR PLASTIC BRACES, and she obviously couldn't count to ten, let alone decipher a receipt. Who did she think she was kidding, clear plastic braces? I could still see them! SOMEONE WAS IN DENIAL.

She listened to most of our story but cut us off short and said something about the ten-dollar store warranty we hadn't bought, and because we hadn't bought it we couldn't get our money back or exchange the disposal for a new one. And the patient and serene Husband with the chubby baby on his chest began spewing obscenities like an eager volcano let loose, his hands on his hips, the dangling innocent baby drooling and smiling at the sparkly plastic braces.

And then he stormed off, huffing and puffing, still uttering obscenity after obscenity, and from behind you could see Leta's arms and legs wiggling as she drooled and cooed and chewed on the collar of her shirt. Why they didn't take us seriously I'LL NEVER KNOW, but all those heaven points we stored up by breastfeeding and sterilizing nipples had just dripped out our leaky disposal.

Later that night a partially ingrown toenail descended upon our household, and I'm not sure there are words that can communicate just how awful was the awfulness of the pain and the ache and the affliction, and did I mention that it was awful? According to sources close to the toenail, the pain shot all the way up from the point of entry, along the shin, around the knee, up up up unto the jawline. Jon's whole body was paralyzed, except for the voice part, which COULD NOT STOP TALKING ABOUT THE PAIN.

This partially ingrown toenail was the most awful partially ingrown toenail there ever was, monumental in its awfulness, and I need to spend the next paragraph talking about just how awful it was, just in case you missed the awfulness that I have already mentioned. It was just so awful, really and very much awful, OH SO AWFUL. And it hurt, and continued to hurt, and in the two seconds since he mentioned it was hurting it hadn't stopped hurting because it still hurt and IT WAS AWFUL.

I know it was just a toe, but it was an important toe. And I understood this, I really did, because my vagina was just a vagina, but it was an important vagina. But he argued that the comparison must stop there because my vagina was designed to stretch and tear like that, but his toe wasn't designed to have the nail part jut into the skin part and it HURT SO BAD. Perhaps if there were stages of pain it would have been more manageable, he said, like how the cervix slowly dilates. At least I had had dilation. The toe doesn't dilate, so the pain in his toe was painful all at once, and this pain had to be talked about, at length, very loudly, with lots of moaning and gnashing of the teeth.

I really wanted to take away his pain, because I didn't like it when he was in pain, but more important, because I would have very much liked to talk about something else. Leta was almost ready to start rolling over! And she could almost touch her face with her foot! And she . . . oh, wait. His toe still hurt. And it was awful. And there was just so much pain.

Did you know that Achilles felt pain, too? In the foot area! And that was not a coincidence. In the middle of moaning about his toe he compared himself to Achilles, and that was just too cute. So I pointed out that Achilles never experienced childbirth, never pushed a swollen

eight-pound rodent out of his vagina and then had to get up and immediately feed that rodent with his breast, so sorry if I am not all that
impressed with Achilles.

Dear Leta,

*Today you turn four months old. I have been trying to keep up
with all the changes going on in your life, but even in the last
twenty-four hours you've learned something new, and I can
only type so fast. This is one of those moments when I wish I
could record you, press pause, and replay you over and over
again so that I don't miss anything. Like when I watch episodes
of reality television and your father makes loud, mean com-
ments, and I have to rewind it to hear what they're saying.*

*A couple of days ago you learned how to blow bubbles and
raspberries with your tongue. This was an inevitable development as you were trying to figure out what to do with all that
drool. Where did you learn to drool like that? We could water
the lawn for a month with all the drool that seeps out of your
mouth on a daily basis. Perhaps all this drool is compensation
for the fact that you never spit up, ever, except for that one
time we were outside talking to the neighbors and you hurled
all over your father's new black business shirt, right after we
had just proudly announced, "She never spits up!" You've got
great timing, kid!*

*You've discovered both of your hands, and they are the most
marvelous creations you have ever seen. You suck on your fingers and then your fist, and sometimes we look over and you*

have both of your thumbs in your mouth, as if one thumb just isn't enough. When we're dressing you for bed at night and we have to pull your pajamas over your arms, you are separated from your hands for all of three seconds, and the look of panic on your face seems to say that you are worried that you will never see them again, oh wonderful hands, come back! And then you are reunited with them, your long-lost friends, and you get so excited that you almost hyperventilate, sticking both fists into your mouth so violently that you almost choke on your knuckles.

This month you also discovered the joy of sticking other things into your mouth. One night a few weeks ago you were lying on your back on our bed and I dangled a teething ring over your head. The room got very quiet, and time seemed to shift into slow motion as you reached up, grabbed the teething ring, opened your mouth, and tried to bring the teething ring to your tongue. But you missed your tongue. You missed your whole mouth altogether and tried to stick the teething ring into your ear. You did this three consecutive times, shoving the teething ring into your ear, and then into your forehead, once into your nose, and then, as the Mormon Tabernacle Choir swelled to a triumphant, room-shaking Hallelujah! you brought the teething ring to your mouth! Fireworks exploded in the distance as you took the teething ring out of your mouth and then put it back in your mouth, over and over again, as if putting that thing in your mouth was what you were born to do. As you squealed in celebration I said good-bye to my old life and hello to my new one, a life that will be consumed with running to grab potentially harmful things out of your hands before they make it to the inside of your eager, drooling jaws.

You are becoming such a little person, and every day I have to resist the urge to put you between two slices of wheat bread and lather mayonnaise on your head, gobbling you up in one bite. Things are so much better, so much more fun now that you have graduated from the oozy, poopy larva stage into an actual baby, one that I can play with, one who responds to my voice and my touch. Your giggles and squeals are delightful, and the once intolerable screaming has been replaced with occasionally hilarious fussiness, thunderous squawks of displeasure as you try to communicate with me that you are mad or angry or just so damn tired of it all! You've never seen a baby so exasperated, and now I have to resist laughing at you because you sound like a really pissed off bird.

A little over a month ago when the screaming was really bad, your father had to come home from work early because I was in a dark, unforgiving place. You had been screaming on and off for hours, and I was crying uncontrollably, still dressed in my pajamas. Your father tried rocking you, singing to you, swinging you. He tried everything I had already tried, and in a moment of frustration he set you down in the crib and walked away to regain some perspective. Twenty seconds later you were asleep. ASLEEP! You fell asleep in twenty seconds and you slept for two hours. That was the beginning of the end of the screaming. It was as if all that screaming was your way of telling us PUT ME DOWN, YOU IDIOTS. Ever since that af-

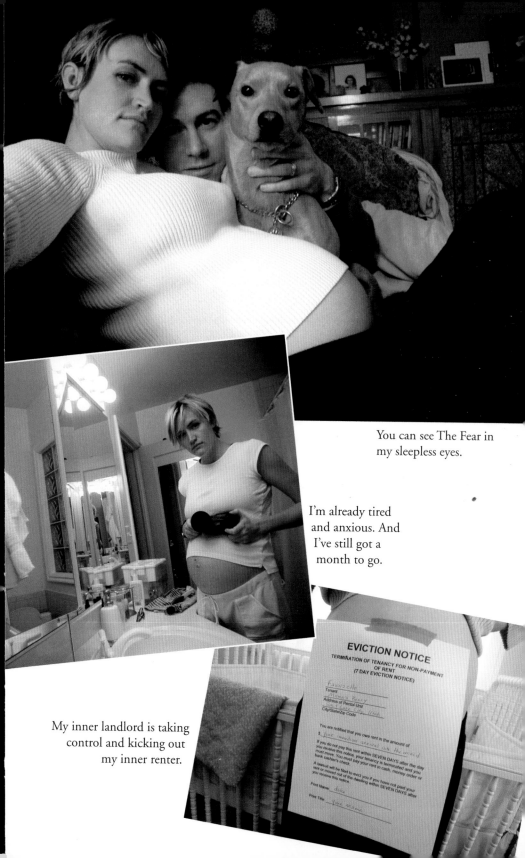

You can see The Fear in my sleepless eyes.

I'm already tired and anxious. And I've still got a month to go.

My inner landlord is taking control and kicking out my inner renter.

EVICTION NOTICE
TERMINATION OF TENANCY FOR NON-PAYMENT OF RENT
(7 DAY EVICTION NOTICE)

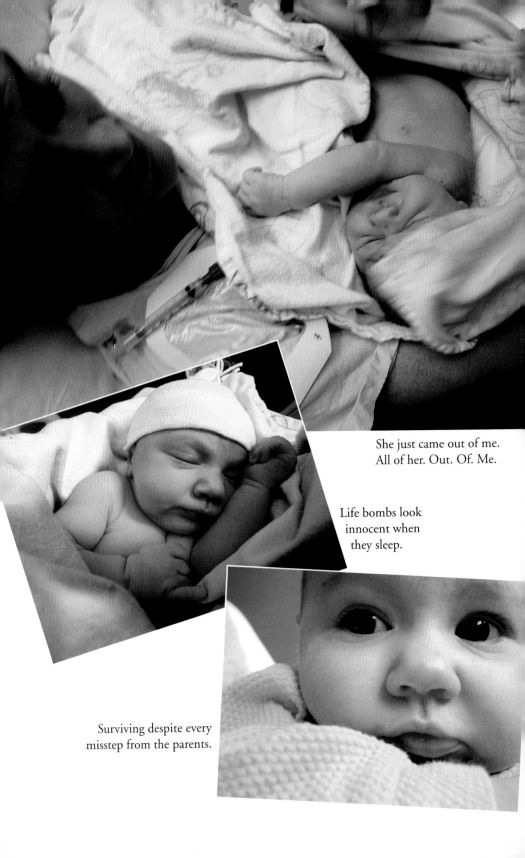

She just came out of me.
All of her. Out. Of. Me.

Life bombs look
innocent when
they sleep.

Surviving despite every
misstep from the parents.

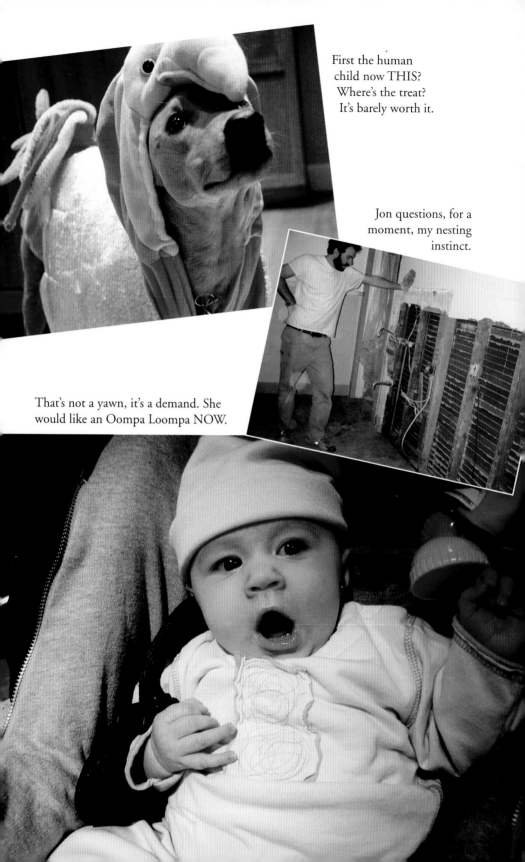

First the human
child now THIS?
Where's the treat?
It's barely worth it.

Jon questions, for a
moment, my nesting
instinct.

That's not a yawn, it's a demand. She
would like an Oompa Loompa NOW.

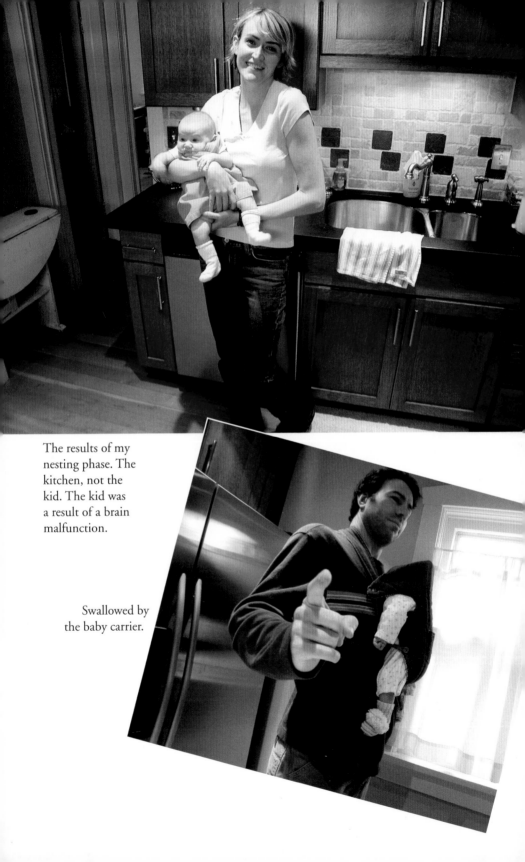

The results of my
nesting phase. The
kitchen, not the
kid. The kid was
a result of a brain
malfunction.

Swallowed by
the baby carrier.

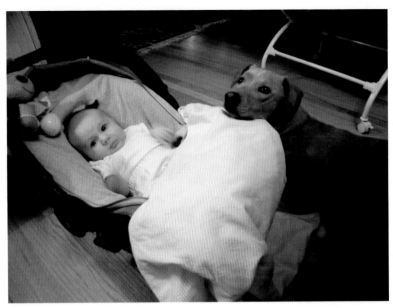

If she's gonna stay, I'll learn to deal with
it. Slowly and begrudgingly.

Manicure courtesy of nerd father who insisted on using the headlamp.
It didn't help.

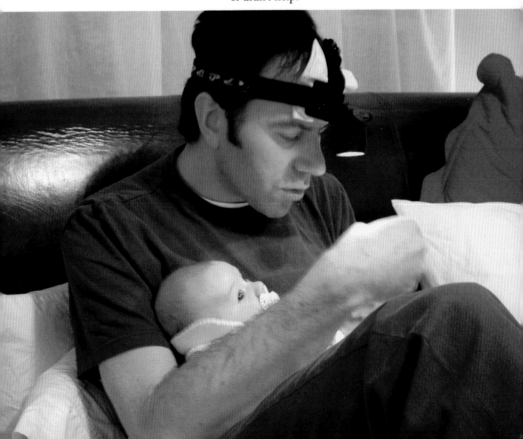

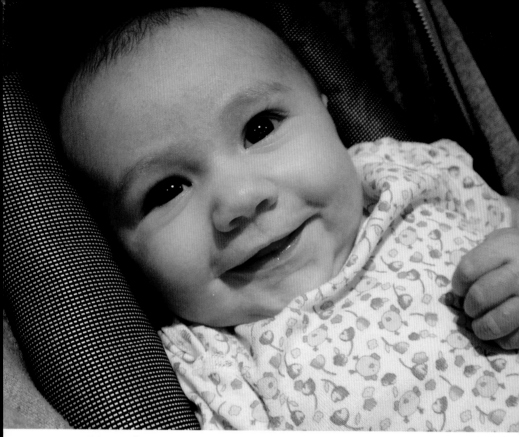

Mama, I love you. Even if I keep you up all night and refuse to be held.

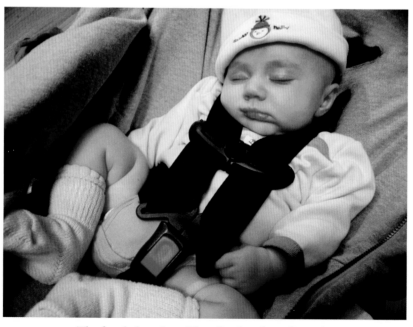

The frog baby asleep. Time for that shot of tequila.

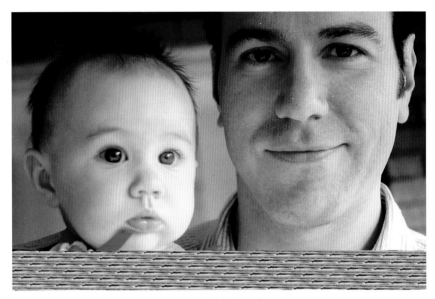

Jon and his "son."

She appears to enjoy cooler weather. She's definitely not my child.

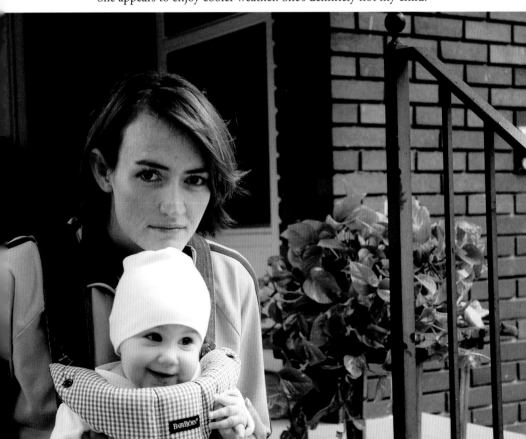

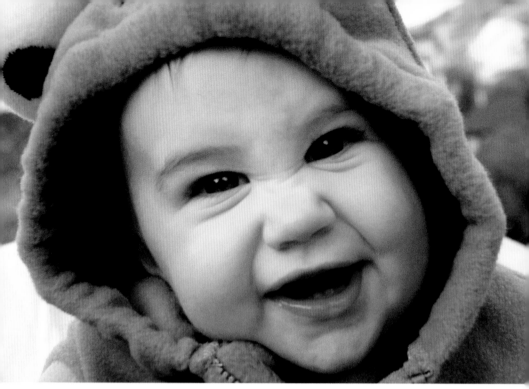

First Halloween! And Mommy's no longer throwing things at Daddy!

If your parents didn't sleep for six straight months they'd look like this, too.

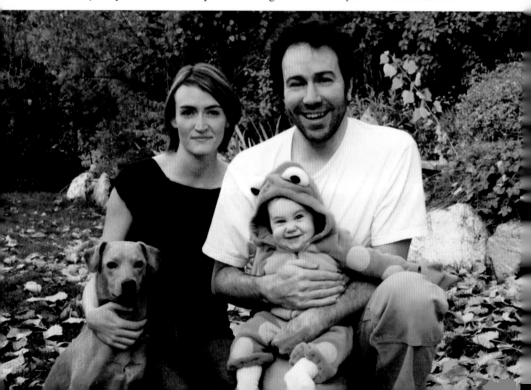

ternoon we put you down in your crib for naps and you fell asleep BY YOURSELF. You don't want to be rocked or sung to or fussed over. In fact, you hate to be fussed over, and if I try to rock you or soothe you to sleep you scream at me. So I leave you alone now when it's time to sleep and you couldn't be happier. THANK YOU, LETA.

I know you're awake when I hear you scratching the mattress. It's your way of letting me know that it's time to come get you, SCRATCH SCRATCH SCRATCH. I can hear the scratching from the most remote point in the house, even outside in the backyard. It's not the prettiest sound, and it makes my spine twitch every time I hear it, but it also breaks my heart it's so damn cute. It's also cute when your father is holding you in the Baby-Björn and you scratch his arm like you scratch the mattress, and then you grab hold of his arm hair and yank it like you're pulling weeds. He shrieks a bit from the sting, but that is okay, because that's his way of sharing in the pain since he didn't have to push you out of his vagina or suffer engorged, torpedo boobs.

Over the weekend you met your Grandpa Hamilton for the first time. He's the man responsible for your pointy chin and the shape of your upper lip, sorry about that. He's a good man though, as good as they come, and you should take his advice when it comes to money and financial planning. However, when he starts talking about politics I want you to cover your ears and kick him in the shins.

What a great month, little one. We are having so much fun together, going on walks and reading books and watching

Pyramid twice a day. Just when I think my love for you couldn't be any bigger, I wake up and discover that I love you even more, and I worry that my body isn't big enough to hold this much love. I worry that my insides may explode because there isn't any more room. I am drunk on my love for you, a sloppy drunk who can't see straight or speak in coherent sentences, a drunk who giggles every time you fart. And it's just so awesome that you're old enough now that you can giggle with me.

Love, Mama

CHAPTER ELEVEN

Other Mothers: Your Harshest Critics

A few days after Leta turned four months old we took away Leta's pacifier and it felt like we were running a division of the Betty Ford Clinic. We'd taken away her cigarettes, her heroin, her daily 64-ounce Diet Coke, and from the resulting hours of weeping and gnashing of the toothless gums you would have thought we'd taken away her will to live.

Our little Robert Downey Jr. cried more in the span of four days than she had in her entire life on earth. She used up all the crying. There was no more crying left in the world. Your baby shouldn't cry anymore because Leta cried enough that week for all the babies ever in the history of mankind and the universe.

Everyone thought we were insane for attempting this intervention, this game of chicken with the most stubborn will ever given a body to enact its wrath. And there were many moments during those days when I wanted to pick up that binky and plug it into her face to stop the wailing, it would have been SO EASY. Maybe a couple of puffs would have tided her over, made the transition a little less painful. But we all know that it would not have stopped at a couple of puffs. She would have wanted those two puffs and then a couple more puffs, and then she would have begged for even more puffs, and within an hour she would have injected the pacifier into her veins.

Once an addict, always an addict. Leta was an abuser.

We probably wouldn't have been in such a hurry to cleanse her of this disease were it not for the terrible things it had done to her sleeping habits, and thus to my sleeping habits, and my sleeping habits took precedence over water and food, over the air that I breathed. Leta needed the pacifier to go to sleep, and when she woke up in the middle of the night and the pacifier wasn't in her mouth she became one pissed infant, like someone had stolen her last pack of cigarettes, the last pack of cigarettes in the world. And for months I'd had to put the binky back in her mouth. I had climbed out of bed, walked into her room, handed her a cigarette and asked, "Do you need a light?"

We'd also discovered that these bad sleeping habits were causing her bad eating habits, and everything could be traced back to the cigarettes: the yellow stains on her fingers, the wrinkles around her lips, the raspy sound of her cough as she swallowed tobacco-colored drool.

All of our problems were tied to that plastic sucking device, and the withdrawal was ripping apart the fragile fabric that held the family together. None of us was sleeping, and both Jon and I developed muscle spasms in our faces and arms. Chuck trembled and licked his empty nut sack every time he heard Leta crying for more binky, and after four days of detox his ass had become a rubbery, hairless knob.

I was on the verge of a mental breakdown. Leta sensed my vulnerability and gave me merciless guilt trips in the form of helpless, wistful gazes that seemed to say, "Mama, why dost thou hurt me so?" And even though I knew I was doing the right thing, that helping her to learn to sleep without the cigarettes would help her eat better and become a healthier, meatier baby that we could sell to the butcher, those gazes pierced my heart and gripped my quivering soul. I knew she was in pain and that she was suffering, and that knowledge was perhaps the worst pain I could endure.

Except for maybe the judgmental snickering of other mothers.

I never knew that the binky was such a political issue, and when we made the decision to cure Leta of her habit we pissed off pretty much every person we knew.

Well-meaning friends informed us that because we had done this to her, Leta was going to suck her thumb until she turned twelve or thirteen years old. Someone even suggested that she'd suck her thumb for the rest of her life and that the only way we'd be able to solve that problem would be to AMPUTATE HER HAND, so I'd better "stop being so mean" and give her back the damn binky.

And then there was the suggestion, repeated over and over my ear, that I let her put the binky back into her mouth herself, duh. Why hadn't I thought of that one myself? Maybe because she was only four months old and possessed the hand-eye coordination of a slug. She could pick up that binky and put it back into her mouth about as well as she could wipe her own ass, and if she was falling behind on that milestone, well then, maybe blame it on all the vodka I fed her in a bottle.

From the sound of the criticism I received you would have thought that Jon and I just woke up one morning and said to each other, "Hey, I've got an idea! Let's take away Leta's pacifier today. It will be a lot of FUN!" Because that's all that kid meant to me, a good time. We'd just take away her soothing mechanism and watch her scream, why not, it would provide hours of laughter and merriment. And let me tell you, I hadn't had that much fun since my OB-GYN took a pair of scissors and sliced a two-inch gash in my vagina. THAT was a fucking riot.

But you know what? Do you want to guess what happened on the fifth night of our intervention? Leta slept for TEN HOURS IN A ROW. TEN. T-E-N.

TEN!!!!!!!!!!!!!!!

That's one, two, three, four, five—wait, I need to catch my breath because there are so many numbers to count . . . phew, okay, that's better, where was I?—six, seven, eight, nine, TEN.

The most Leta had ever slept up until that night was six hours in a row, and that was just a side effect of her two-month immunizations. It only happened once, and since that night the longest she had ever slept in a row was three hours. Taking away her binky tripled her sleeping capacity. That can't be a bad thing, right? Oh wait, I forgot. If my baby slept that long that meant I was neglecting her. I'd never learn!

Guess what else happened? No, guess. GUESS!!

She started eating! During the day! In the daytime! When it was day outside! MY BABY KNEW HOW TO EAT, WHY HAD NO ONE TOLD ME?

But just because Leta slept ten hours, however, didn't mean that I slept any of those hours, any at all whatsoever. I woke up every hour and half hour waiting for the wailing, my heart clinched up in my throat. And then it got later and later, and the wailing never came, and when she finally woke up (TEN HOURS LATER! REMEMBER?), my boobs were so full I could have sprayed milk twenty feet into the air. I hopped out of bed, two rock hard concrete traffic mounds on my chest, and ran to my binky-less Wonderchild, attaching her to my boob before I even had her out of the crib. She could barely keep up with the flow, my boob a gushing fire hydrant that she was trying to stop with her mouth.

On Father's Day I got a little weepy, a little carried away in my emotion for the man who'd given my daughter the blueprint for her DNA. Our child inherited his eyes and his nose, his profile and his forehead, and pretty much everything else. I could not look at her without seeing him.

I often felt that parenthood seemed lopsided. Mothers were the ones who had to suffer all sorts of unimaginable pain to bring the child into the world while the father got to sit to the side, smoke cigars, and pat the kid on the butt from time to time. And while that wasn't an entirely accurate depiction of our roles in Leta's life, it was a pretty accurate depiction of the intrinsic nature of this process.

Becoming a mother had been very hard for me. My pregnancy was marked with nausea and bloating and swelling and thirty pounds of weight gain and heartburn and insomnia and a never-ending need to go pee. Labor wasn't so bad, if you can say such a thing about that kind of pain, it being "not so bad." I was fortunate in that I didn't experience any complications, but the aftermath was Biblical in its devastation.

There were stitches and chronic constipation and crying and hemorrhoids and bladder infections and back pains and bleeding and crying and cracked nipples and crying and lumpy breasts with the texture and firmness of granite. And then there were weeks and weeks of crying and sleep deprivation and depression and anxiety and hard, hard, uncomfortable breasts.

Jon got to share in the sleep deprivation, but his main physical contribution to bringing this baby into the world, aside from his Very Potent Sperm, was carrying me every step of the way. He hadn't experienced any of the physical pain of the process, but he had picked me up off the floor more times than was required under the law for men who were married to Really Difficult Women.

He held my head when I puked; he cheered for me when I tried to pee. He helped me turn over in the middle of the night when I was so whalelike in size that I couldn't turn over by myself.

He pushed with me during labor and almost passed out from depriving his brain of oxygen. He changed Leta's first diaper even though we both hadn't slept in forty-eight hours, and the diapers in the hospital were all broken, and the meconium stuck to every pore in his forearm.

He stood outside the door when I went to poop for the first time after labor, The Most Horrible Day of My Life, coaching me like I was going through labor again, giving birth to Leta's twin. And then he held my head as I cried afterward.

He had come home from work early (more times than I was proud to admit) to wipe away my tears, to calm the baby's screaming as I screamed in the other room.

He rubbed my feet because he wanted to, not because I asked him to. He let me sleep an extra thirty minutes in the morning at least three or four times a week because he knew that those extra minutes were the key to my sanity.

He let me spew nonsense every night, and then he let me cry and cry some more. And then he held me once again.

And then there was his relationship with Leta.

Jon put Leta to bed every night. When I saw them together in the rocking chair reading stories together, sharing those quiet evening moments, father and daughter, my heart would break into a million pieces.

I think about how he could have chosen someone else. He could have looked at me across that table years ago and said, "You are nice and all, but I need to see other women." He could have walked out of my life any number of times. He could have given another woman a child with his eyes.

But there he was, my husband, Leta's father. He had endured pain he never knew he would have to endure at the hands of my disease, and he stood by me, carried me through many sleepless nights. His contribution was as vital as mine.

The best part of my day was when Jon carried Leta back to the changing table after her bath, and she'd lay there wrapped in the towel, her hand shoved as far as she could get it into the back of her mouth. He'd lean down and pretend to eat her neck, causing her to laugh. And she laughed for him like she laughed for no one else, a full-body laugh that shook her belly and caused her to let go of her hand for a second. Her giggles would fill the house and echo through the baby monitor into the living room and out to the street. I imagined that those echoing giggles were what the background music in heaven sounded like.

The first time we fed Leta solid food she smeared the entire jar all over her face, and three days later we were still finding sweet potatoes in her ears. I don't know why they call it solid because there was nothing solid about it. If it had been solid then she wouldn't have been able to paint with it, and she used her whole body as her canvas.

I'll be honest and admit that I thought it was going to be easy to feed a baby. I was just going to shove a little bit of food into her mouth and she'd swallow it like a reasonable human being. She stuck everything else into her mouth, so wouldn't she be delighted that this particular thing actually had taste! A sweet taste! Not at all bitter like the paper towels she'd snatch out of my hands and shove down her throat!

But how many times have I seen pictures of babies with food smeared all over their faces? I always thought that parents smeared the food on the baby's face because babies are cute with mushy vegetables on their foreheads. Who doesn't love a baby with carrots dripping from her nostrils? That's a perk of parenthood, getting to decorate one's baby with colorful foodstuffs and then taking a picture and posting it on the Internet, right? But the baby SELF-DECORATES, I did not know this, and the mess from this self-decoration becomes exponentially worse by the second as it travels from spoon to face to hand to everything within a two-mile radius. Two days after we fed Leta sweet potatoes they found some splattered all over the gates of the Mormon temple downtown.

I had to take the idiocy one step further and carry out this experiment on our couch. Our custom-made, blue velvet, imported down-filled couch. And in the panic of the moment I couldn't think straight, and instead of doing the thinking-straight thing and running to get wipes to salvage our couch and our coffee table and the refinished hardwood floors, I did the non-thinking-straight thing which seemed like the thinking-straight thing at the time. I began LICKING UP THE SWEET POTATOES WITH MY TONGUE, starting with her face.

That was the fun part.

I licked her cheeks and her nose, then her hands and wrists, and then I ate her chin, and then her third and fourth chin. This did nothing to alleviate the mess. It did, however, taste very sweet, and I walked around for a week with a faint orange tattoo of a small hand on my forehead.

LESSON CONCERNING SOLID FOOD: learned.

In the weeks leading up to Leta's birth I received several gifts from friends, including infant clothing and receiving blankets, breast pads and tiny nail clippers. I remember looking at all the stuff and wondering, "What the hell do you do with a breast pad? Can you eat these things?" because I had no idea what I was getting myself into. I honestly thought that the baby would come with all the clothes she needed. After giving birth to the baby and the placenta, I thought a whole package of cotton onesies would shoot out the birth canal, followed closely by several nightgowns and a six-pack of tiny pink socks. I had gained so much weight that I was certain Leta would arrive with luggage.

I'd learned a lot in the few months since I had been a parent. I'd learned that babies don't necessarily like to be dangled by their toes from the rooftop or to have their mouths clamped shut with clothespins. Duct tape worked better at silencing the screaming than swings or strollers or diaper changes. I'd also become an expert on the subject of breast pads (no, you cannot eat those things), and could shoot breast milk at a target thirty feet away.

Every night Jon and I took inventory of what we'd learned and added it to our notebook of parenting: Leta did not like to be outside; she did not like the vacuum cleaner or other obnoxious noises; she liked the book about the ladybug, but not the book about the rocking horse; Leta would stop screaming if I sang a certain Morrissey song, but I couldn't sing it in my normal voice and had to instead imitate Morrissey because she knew the difference.

And finally: Leta would use solid food to draw intricate landscapes on our expensive furniture.

Dear Leta,

Today you turn five months old. FIVE! WHOLE! MONTHS! You're practically an adult! Isn't it about time you started paying rent?

The first thing we should talk about is how you've slept through the night five nights in a row. And when I say slept through the night I don't mean six or seven hours in a row. Six or seven hours is for three-month-olds, for babies. When I say slept through the night I mean twelve HOURS IN A ROW, from 7 PM until 7 AM. You're sleeping better than most Harvard graduates, Leta.

You have discovered the joy of sleeping, something you definitely inherited from me. Your naps are now all an hour or longer, sometimes even two hours. And when we put you in the crib for a nap, you smile, bring your fist to your mouth, and close your eyes. When you wake up in the morning you usually lie in the crib for five to ten minutes just playing with your blankets and examining your abnormally large hands, waiting for us to come get you. And when we come get you it's like you're playing the slots and have just hit JACKPOT! Your whole body convulses with excitement and you gasp and smile and squint your forehead with glee! The look on your face seems to say THERE IS THAT WOMAN WHO FEEDS ME! or THERE IS THAT MAN WHO MAKES ME LAUGH ALL THE TIME!

And since we're talking about the laughing . . . you have this low, back-of-the-throat laugh that sounds like a fake laugh. Sometimes it sounds like you are laughing to make us feel good about our attempts to make you laugh, like, "Haha, I know you're trying to be funny, but you're really not that funny, and since I don't want you to feel bad I'll just go ahead and laugh anyway, you sad, pathetic people." It sounds so fake that I always expect you to roll your eyes.

But then there are the full-bodied chuckles that only your father can seem to elicit from you, and every time he makes you chuckle, open-mouthed and wide-eyed, he gives you the hiccups. This wouldn't normally be a problem except that it always happens right before bedtime. So the whole time I'm feeding you dinner you're hiccuping, and the hiccups continue throughout your bedtime story. Sometimes the hiccups don't stop until about ten minutes after you've fallen asleep, so you sound like a beer-bellied frat boy who has passed out after drinking two cases of Old Milwaukee.

So you're sleeping well and laughing and being a cute little kid all around, but there is something we need to talk about: why must you make that awful noise when you are bored? Why can't you be patient and quiet and lovable when you're just sitting there, instead of going, "Iiiiiiiiiiiihhhhh! Iiiiiiiiiiiiihhhhh!!" like a sick and diseased goat who has been left by the herd on the side of a mountain to be gobbled up by wolves?

I live my life in two-hour increments. Once you wake in the morning or from a nap I have to come up with distracting activities to fill the two hours until you go down for your next nap, otherwise you bleat, not out of discomfort or pain, but out of anger and disappointment at being left all alone in the room, except not really all alone because I'm sitting there RIGHT BESIDE YOU. If we aren't engaged in a new activity with new toys you haven't seen before, you assault me with the most annoying noise ever uttered in the universe. So we go on walk after walk after walk, and then we go to the grocery store, and then to the park, and then we read books and play with rattles and spoons and measuring cups, and that's just the first fifteen minutes. After two hours of nonstop Project

Distraction, I'm ready to collapse from exhaustion, and you seem only slightly amused as if you're thinking, "Is this the best that you can do?"

This month you have learned how to reach for things, which is rather unfortunate because you haven't yet learned how to balance yourself, so anytime you reach for something you end up face first on the floor or the couch. Surprisingly, this isn't nearly as frustrating as being bored (bleat! bleat!), and you could remain in the face-plant position for several minutes without announcing any sort of discomfort. I don't know if that's because you trust me to come running to your rescue or because you're studying the pattern on the floor and want to be left alone in your research.

Also, this month I have gone on a carb-only diet consisting of orange juice, strawberry Pop-Tarts, and your chubby cheeks. I cannot keep your face out of my mouth, it is just so scrumptious and plump and chewy and round. You have a lot more hair on your head, so instead of putting your whole head in my mouth I bite off your ears and nose and gnaw on your chin. And then I go back for more cheeks. Sometimes I just can't stop and I end up swallowing you whole and I walk around with your feet hanging out of my mouth. When your father comes home from work he asks, "Where's the baby?" And I have to confess, "I ate her."

Love, Mama

CHAPTER TWELVE

Trusting the Wisdom of a Dog

*N*ever underestimate the importance of a mutual love and need for wiper fluid within a marriage. How many families are being torn apart because one spouse doesn't understand the value of a clean windshield while the other spouse cannot breathe air knowing that the windshield is dirty?

When I was single I broke up with men because they refused to wash their windshields. One of them claimed that it just wasn't dirty enough, and that he would be wasting wiper fluid if he went ahead and cleaned the windshield, as if there aren't hundreds of thousands of bottles of wiper fluid sitting idly at every supermarket and auto parts store in the world WAITING TO BE BOUGHT AND USED TO CLEAN WINDSHIELDS. So he would drive around with all this shit on his windshield—bird poop and water stains and mud and various other fluids of curious origin—and he could barely see out of a two-inch space *on the passenger side of the window.* We argued about the state of his windshield incessantly. I refused to go anywhere in his car because I would have to sit there looking at the filth, and I would want to throw up and punch him. So we broke up, partly because of the windshield, partly because he had this other habit of being a homosexual.

If I'm not careful I can go through a couple of gallons of wiper fluid a week. I clean the windshield every time I get into the car, and then three or four times while I'm driving city streets, a couple dozen times if I'm on the freeway. There is just no reason to drive around with crap on the windshield, not when you can pull back that lever and hear the heavenly gush of wiper fluid, oh cleansing baptismal blue liquid! The power! To clean the windshield of the car WHILE THE CAR IS IN MOTION!

Is there a worse sound in the world than the coughing, dry clanking of an empty wiper fluid reservoir? And then the immediate, echoing realization that the sacred pools of cleanser have dried up and that you might have to drive a whole mile with bird poop in the middle of your line of sight? The horror! Let me gouge out my eyes with forks rather than drive another inch without my wiper fluid!

My marriage is built upon a mutual understanding of the hallowed nature of wiper fluid. The first time I saw him reach for that lever to cleanse the windshield I knew that he was a keeper. Imagine my squealing delight when he continued to hold that lever back for TEN WHOLE SECONDS. He doesn't just clean his windshield; he *showers* it with love.

Sometimes Leta and I would sit on the porch in the mornings to watch Jon pull out of the driveway and turn up the street to go to work. Invariably I would watch as the morning sun reflected in rainbow sheets off the shooting waterfalls of wiper fluid as he cleaned the windshield near the corner of our block. I liked to think of it as his way of waving good-bye, bidding me a good day, one he hoped was full of clean windshields.

My mother and I were sitting at a restaurant having lunch when we both noticed that Leta was trying to put the table in her mouth. The whole table. We could see the concentration in her face, her thoughts swarming around how she could pull the whole table closer and fit it in her mouth. She had already burned through every toy I had packed in my purse (her response to each toy was, "You're joking, right? I have already seen this toy before, therefore it possesses no entertainment value. You obviously aren't trying hard enough, and now I must scream."), plus six or seven packets of sugar that she would suck and then violently discard by throwing them at the person sitting next to us. We had only begun our appetizers, and the level of Leta's boredom had reached Terror Level: RUN FOR YOUR LIVES.

Rarely did I get to have lunch with my mother. She worked in Los Angeles five days a week, and on the weekends she had to split her time among forty family members whose sole purpose in life was to make her feel guilty. Sometimes she'd stop by our house on the way to or from the airport so that she could snack on Leta's cheeks, but then she'd be off again having spoken only a few words to me, those words being "hello," "good-bye," or "Where's that baby?"

That particular lunch, however, lasted four hours and was the longest amount of time I had spent with my mother in *years*. This can be explained by the fact that I hadn't been that depressed in years, or ever, and I finally decided to risk being one of those forty demanding family members and told her that I needed help. I needed help because I was on the edge, and I was holding on to that edge with my fingertips, my body dangling precariously over a dark hole that was reaching up to swallow me.

I kept thinking that my depression would go away, that my self-medication was going to work. But I should have known better than anyone else that this just doesn't go away. In fact, it festered and grew until one morning I found myself throwing things in the general direction of loving and wonderful people who did not deserve to have things thrown in their general direction. It had entered my bloodstream and was systematically choking me to death.

Leta was sleeping unbelievably well, and I hadn't had to feed her during the night in over ten days. But I had't slept any of those nights. I lay awake at night waiting for her call, waiting for something to go wrong, waiting for someone to take her away from me. I couldn't sleep thinking about how *I* wouldn't want to come home to me, why did Jon continue to come home to me?

I'd get up in the morning having slept only an hour or two and couldn't imagine living another minute. The expanse of the day unfolded before me and I couldn't comprehend how I was going to distract my cranky baby for the next twelve hours. There'd be walks and more walks and books and rattles and moving from the porch to the sidewalk and back to the porch to delay her disappointment just a few more minutes. And then there were the moments when I couldn't do anything to stop her from screaming at me, and it felt like she was sad that she didn't have a mother who knew what the hell she was doing.

I used to be sad only in the morning, and after 11 AM I was okay. But the mornings started to turn into afternoons, then into nights, and soon it got to the point that I was never okay. There wasn't a moment in the day that I looked forward to. I didn't see an end to this cycle of stress, and I found myself asking much too often, "Why go on?"

I finally saw a psychiatrist who prescribed me a new combination of drugs, ones completely different from the ones I had been trying. I wished that there were other ways that I could have gone about getting better, but I knew that what I was feeling was beyond the help of herbal remedies or dietary changes. I exercised all the time and I had a very healthy diet, but my situation had become life-threatening. I was truly afraid that I would hurt myself.

Slowly I started taking an antianxiety drug and a mood stabilizer, two very powerful drugs that had to be monitored. The doctor did not prescribe a sleep aid because he thought that the antianxiety drug would stop the incessant and unnecessary worrying that kept me awake at night. I felt very positive about this, hopeful that the drugs would work and that I would one day soon be able to wake up in the morning and recognize what a wonderful life I had.

But there was one terrible drawback to the step I was taking toward sanity. The doctor told me that I would have to wean Leta if I wanted to work up to therapeutic levels of these drugs. I'd have to stop breast-feeding in the next month.

I never thought that I would feel so devastated at the prospect of having to stop breastfeeding. I couldn't talk about it without crying. I really believed that feeding Leta was the only way that she was comforted by me, and once that was gone would she even know who I was?

The strange thing was that breastfeeding had never been the beautiful and peaceful and wondrous endeavor that they wanted me to believe it was. I'm sure it had been for many women, but for me it had been a struggle from the first moment she latched on in the hospital. It started out with excruciating pain, and then continued being painful for a month, and then five months later I still got engorged when she didn't eat a full meal. And Leta didn't *ever* eat a full meal, so I was constantly worried about whether or not she was getting enough to eat.

I tried pumping for a few weeks, but every time I pumped I got a clog in my left boob and spent several days afterward hunched over in paralyzing pain. I couldn't count how many nights I lay in bed awake waiting for her to wake up so that she would eat and the pain in my chest could subside for at least a few hours.

There had been moments, a select few moments when feeding her was an almost religious experience. Moments when she'd stop eating, smile, and reach her hand up to touch my face. My beautiful baby in my arms so close to my chest, her soft fingers exploring the line of my chin. Those were moments when I believed in God.

But I knew that if I didn't stop breastfeeding I would be doing the selfish thing. I understood that. I understood that I had to get better for the sake of my family, and I believed that the drugs were my only hope. But I didn't think my heart could break into so many pieces. I didn't know how much I loved feeding my baby, how fundamental it had been to my relationship with her, how much I had sacrificed to continue breastfeeding. My God, I didn't want to give it up.

So one afternoon I let myself cry for hours about it, and usually when I cried Chuck would scurry out of the room to get as far away from me as possible. But that afternoon he sat on top of me, his face pressed up into my armpit, trying to get as close to me as possible. I think he knew that I needed him. I imagined he was trying to tell me, "You didn't breastfeed me, and look how awesome I turned out." And then he would say, "It's going to be okay."

And I believed him.

But first, there were other indignities to endure, ones that would make me question just who the hell I had become.

Leta's first extended car trip was a two-hour ride through the desert to some property my mother had recently bought in Duchesne, Utah. For those of you who like myself tend to pronounce words the way they are spelled, you would be wrong in assuming that Duchesne is pronounced Doo-chez-nee. The correct pronunciation is Doo-Shane, and should be uttered as if your front two teeth are missing because you were never taught proper hygiene while growing up in your double-wide down by the river.

So we all piled into my mother's Mormon Mobile—a car large enough to hold twenty-two children from three different wives that had enough space left over to pick up a fourth wife down at the local middle school—and headed out at about eight o'clock on a bright July morning. Occupants of the car included my mother, my stepfather, my sister, my brother-in-law, Grumpelstiltskin, and myself. The trip to Doo-chez-nee was two hours one way.

I had warned everyone that Leta didn't do so well when she couldn't sleep in her crib, but they all assured me that she would have no problems falling asleep in her car seat, as if I hadn't spent the last five months of my life witnessing just how badly Leta slept in her car seat.

Babies are supposed to take naps during the day, which can sometimes be bothersome if you want to live a thing called life. When babies don't nap they can become cranky and unbearable, and they send you subliminal messages that say PLEASE THROW ME OUT THE NEAREST WINDOW. Leta took three, fifteen-second catnaps in the car during our eight-hour round trip to Doo-chez-nee, for a whopping total of forty-five seconds of sleep. Her subliminal messages to me talked about the window and the throwing, but they were specific about which window and that window was the one on the passenger side of the moving vehicle.

She was not happy. And no amount of yummy teething biscuits or rattles or soothing rubbing of the infant feet could calm her down. Again, she did all of the screaming for all of the babies in the world and continued to do so even when my beautiful, tan sister tried to comfort her. My baby could not be comforted by a beautiful, tan, flaxen-haired babe with big boobs. WHAT WAS WRONG WITH MY CHILD?

In the middle of the trip we stopped at a greasy burger joint in Roosevelt, Utah, so that the other members of my family could eat hamburgers WITHOUT THE BUNS, because they're on That Diet. I had to sit in the car for several minutes so that I could feed Leta, and in the middle of the feeding she shit neon orange poop out the back of her infant jeans and up to her shoulder blades. It was the type of poop that could glow in the dark, one that required a fire hose to clean up. Since it was blisteringly hot I did something that I promised myself I would never do: I left her in nothing but her diapers and socks and went into a public establishment. And she looked like a hobo baby.

Not surprisingly, my shirtless baby was the most civilized creature in that restaurant, as everyone there looked related, in the sense that everyone seemed like brothers or uncles or BOTH AT THE SAME TIME. That didn't stop my Grumpling Wonder from grabbing hold of my large Sprite and tossing it to the floor in a thundering explosion that left the floors, walls, tables, and neighboring counties covered in carbonated stickiness.

Was that really me? Had I gone that far? Was I really carrying around a sticky, shirtless baby? At least she had socks on!

The last thirty minutes of the drive home were perhaps the most horrible thirty minutes of my mother's and sister's lives as Leta, sitting between them, screamed at the top of her lungs all the way from Park City to our neighborhood. My mother asked me if I understood her different screams and what this one could possibly mean, and for the first time in my life I didn't hesitate at dropping The Mother in front of my mother and I said, "Leta is saying, 'GET ME THE FUCK OUT OF THIS CAR.' " And then my mother said, "Well, I guess she means business."

During Leta's fifth month of life we spent an entire day at various government institutions renewing my driver's license and procuring Leta's birth certificate. I was supposed to get my driver's license renewed the week we moved to Utah almost a year previously, but doing so would have been lawful and responsible, and I'd left that church a long time ago. Plus, the picture on my California license was one of the only pictures of me that I actually liked, one in which you couldn't really tell that my left eye drooped more than my right eye, and the look on my face seemed to scream YOU PEOPLE HAVE NO IDEA HOW STUPID YOU ARE TO LET ME OPERATE A VEHICLE.

I just want to point out that I aced the Utah written driver's test. It was the old anal-retentive valedictorian in me clawing its way out. Forget about the fact that the test was open book, and that the book had a table of contents that said, "The answer to question #5 can be found on page 42." I don't want to point out that I failed the California written driver's test four times, and that the only way I actually got my license was to promise my firstborn child to the enormous Latina woman giving the test. I had no doubt that Leta would lead a long, fulfilling life once I stuck her in a UPS box and shipped her to Torrance, CA, where she would remain under the watchful eye of an enormous Latina woman and her friends at the California DMV. Sorry, kid! Mama had to drive!

The kind people at Delta Air Lines informed us that if we ever intended to fly with Leta we needed to have her birth certificate in order to prove that she was under twenty-four months old, which made sense considering that Leta sometimes looked like a balding sixty-four-year-old plumber from Bucksnort, Tennessee, and God knows he shouldn't be allowed to sit in anyone's lap. We spent the better part of the afternoon standing in line at the Department of Health in the company of the Dregs of Humanity, people who hadn't bathed since Reagan left office. More than a few women were wearing house slippers and pink curlers in their matted hair, unaware that they had gotten out of bed, left the house, and were standing in public.

Jon and I seemed to be the only people in the room who still had our original teeth, and just when I couldn't feel more high and mighty about how much better of a person I was than these stinky, primal swamp monsters, my baby started throwing things ACROSS. THE. ROOM. None of the other swamp babies were throwing things, but my baby—the baby of two educated and recently showered parents— refused to keep the toy in her hand and insisted upon projecting the toy with much latitudinal oomph at innocent and polite swamp people. I may have been the only woman in the room wearing clean underwear, but I was also the only woman in the room whose kid needed to be duct taped into submission. Is there any force more equalizing and humbling than parenthood?

• • •

On the morning of Leta's last breastfed meal she slept in a half hour later than usual, so I lay there awake waiting for her morning noises, little grunts and sighs and gurgles that say, "Please come get me now because I am awake and very, very cute."

I tried not to think about how that morning was going to be the last time I would ever breastfeed her, but of course that's *all* I could think about. Both of my boobs were leaking, and the pain of not feeding in over twelve hours was settling in my chest and making its way up to my neck. I secretly wished that she would remain sleeping all day, perhaps forever, so that we would never have to have a last feeding. Sometimes I felt this way about her developmental stages, like why did she have to grow teeth? Couldn't she be gummy forever? Life could be lived without teeth, just ask my Granny. And crawling? Crawling is so overrated. It's hard on the knees.

I'd been bound to this child for six months without any break, and that morning as she snuggled in my arms and ate her last boob-delivered breakfast I sobbed and gushed tears on her porcelain soft cheeks. And when she was full I held her close a few extra minutes so that she could lift her arm to my face and pinch my nose. And then I put her whole hand in my mouth to nibble on her fat fingers and to muffle my weeping.

I won't ever forget the way she constantly moved her hands and feet while she ate, grabbing at my shirt and scratching the Holy Living Shit out of the back of my arm. She would use whichever hand was free to pound my chest, or to seek out my face, or to stick straight up in the air like an empty flagpole. Sometimes she would cup her face or her head and sigh as if to say, "God, this job is hard, but somebody's gotta do it, I guess." And I'd always respond, "Leta, there are children somewhere in Africa right now who would LOVE a clean boob to suck on."

In the weeks leading up to that morning she had become easily distracted while eating and would stop mid-suck to see who else was in the room or to study the pattern on the pillowcase or to scream at me because I was watching *Pyramid* without her. One afternoon I was feeding her on the couch while cleaning off the TiVo hard drive, and I started an episode of *Pyramid*. The moment she heard Donny Osmond's insipid, robotic clucking her eyes got as big as hubcaps and she stopped eating, whipped her head around, and stiffened her body like a plank of wood, a recent trick of hers to signal TOTAL AND UTTER DISSATISFACTION, as if the CONSTANT, INCESSANT, NEVERENDING BLEATING wasn't getting the point across already. How could I watch our favorite game show while she was facing the other way, oh horrible, mean and unloving beast-mother?

I'd received a lot of advice about drugs and breastfeeding and weighing my options and making sure that I wasn't weaning unnecessarily, but I knew it was something I had to do, and although it was ripping me apart inside I actually felt comforted at having made the choice. I believed that this was the first step toward me getting better, toward me remaining alive and not leaving my daughter without a mother, or leaving my husband without a companion or lover.

Leta spent the next three days with my mother, who got her to take the bottle on her very first try, even though I had warned her that she would be dealing with the most stubborn force in the universe, more powerful than gravity, more toxic than nuclear radiation; she'd be tending Leta, God's Revenge. And every night when she was returned to me she acted like a totally different kid. She'd sit there like normal babies just sit there, making normal baby sounds, sounds that weren't goatlike or torturous. And her smiles were even bigger than before! HUGE SMILES. It was like she was so goddamned relieved that she didn't have to suck on that stupid tit anymore.

Dear Leta,

You turn six months old in a few days. I would normally wait until the actual day of your six month mark to write this, but we're going to be at a family reunion all week and my hands will most likely be tied behind my back so that I don't CHOKE ANYONE TO DEATH.

Six months. Good gravy, child. That's as long as the same-as-cash financing plan on our warshing machine. Yes, that's right. Your mother pronounces washing as warshing, and SO WILL YOU. Your father may try to convince you otherwise, but crayon is pronounced as crown, ruin as ru-een, and iron as arn. Speaking this way will endear you to others and will also beguile and distract anyone in law enforcement who is giving you a hard time. Remember this, Leta, when the DNA governing your driving skills kicks in and you find yourself trying to outrun Utah Highway Patrol after a hard night of partying in Park City: the key is to stretch every single-syllable word into three or more distinct syllables. Oh, and showing some cleavage works, too.

This month you have spent most of your waking hours grabbing things and shoving them into your mouth. There is nothing in this world off-limits to your grabbing and eating. You've gobbled other people's hair, the wireless phone antenna, ce-

ramic drink coasters, the dog's tail, and both of your feet AT THE SAME TIME.

I'll never forget the first time you took hold of your right foot and pulled it to your mouth. You were lying on the changing table getting prepped for bed, and you snatched up that foot like you were stealing food off someone else's plate. And then you stuck it in your mouth, and the stunned look on your face seemed to say, "What is this? A third hand? To chew on? You mean I have three hands? Why have you been hiding this from me, this third hand to chew on?" I could see the cogs in your brain clicking and clacking as you suddenly realized that if there was a third hand, THERE JUST MIGHT BE A FOURTH ONE AROUND HERE SOMEWHERE! And there you were, my chubby, naked baby contorted like a pretzel on the changing table, all limbs of your body in your mouth. You looked up at me as if to say, "This, this is the American dream."

Last week you spent three days with Grandmommy who introduced you to a bottle and to the joys of artificially flavored suckers. She would return you home every night before bed and I honestly thought that she had returned the wrong baby. Something changed when you started taking the bottle, something wonderful happened. It was as if we had unmasked A BABY! You've been WONDROUS this week, making all these happy noises and smiling and laughing your ass off. Where have you been? Why have you been hiding from me?

Sadly and tragically the bottle has also changed the substance that comes out of your hind section. For six months you were exclusively breastfed and the poop that came out of your butt was just a liquid that sometimes possessed an interesting color and texture. It never had an offensive odor. But now, now that you're taking formula and eating food, that inoffensive liquid has turned into ACTUAL HUMAN FECES. You have SHIT coming out of your ASS! And I have to clean it up! With my HANDS! I am having a hard time reconciling the fact that my precious punkin buttercup could manufacture something so foul and revolting. You no longer poop in your diaper. Now . . . now you crap your pants.

This month I also got you to fall asleep on my shoulder, FOR THE VERY FIRST TIME. It was no small feat, and I had to walk up and down the length of our house and sing Morrissey OUT LOUD ("America, you know where you can shove your hamburger!"), but you eventually gave in to the exhaustion and passed out in the curve of my neck. That was one of the most beautiful moments of my life, having you there motionless and heavy from sleep, the smell of your powder-fresh head smeared across my cheek.

Leta, you are so lovely. You have made my life so complex and crazy and intense, but recently I have been waking up really early and counting the minutes until you wake up. I get so excited to see those Armstrong eyes and that Hamilton chin, and I want to rush in and ask you if you want to play. I'll hold your feet while you eat them!

Love, Mama

P.S. You rolled over today! TWICE! And then immediately looked up at us like "WHAT THE FUCK JUST HAPPENED?"

CHAPTER THIRTEEN

Finally, Proof That I Was in the Room When She Was Conceived

A few days after Leta turned six months old we packed up the entire house and spent the next four days in the mountains with my side of the family, a raucous group of people that includes my sister and her five kids, my brother and his three kids, my mother and stepfather, and my stepfather's bologna. My mother thought it would be fun for all of us to spend ninety-six hours in a small cabin with no air-conditioning at an altitude so uncomfortable that it regularly squeezed out the oil from my teenage niece's pimples.

I was surprisingly excited about this trip if only because I would be getting a much needed break from the minute-to-minute upkeep of the wee one. On the first morning of this retreat we joined the entire family for a short hike just a few miles away from our cabin. This decision was a big step for me because the hike would interfere with Leta's sleeping schedule, and I was a bit of a stickler when it came to Leta's sleeping schedule. Interference caused screaming. Have I ever told you about the screaming? I don't know if I have ever mentioned the screaming, but in case I haven't this is all you need to know: You wouldn't have liked Leta when she screamed.

The previous day Leta had taken three thirty-minute catnaps, and that was all the napping she did for the entire day. It was partly her fault because she was very stubborn and found her mama's anxiety attacks somewhat amusing. But her catnaps were also the result of the family in the cabin directly next to ours, a family who thought it was perfectly normal to rev their ATVs all day long outside our window. If that family was missing their sixteen-year-old son who had a bad attitude and needed to stand up straight and button up his shirt, the sixteen-year-old kid who based his entire self-worth on how loud he could gun that engine, I can honestly say that I MOST CERTAINLY DID NOT strangle him and throw him in the river.

So I woke up Wednesday and thought to myself, why am I sitting around this cabin being held prisoner by an unbuttoned sixteen-year-old? And when Leta woke up I informed her, "It's your turn to work around MY schedule, and we are going to go on this hike and you are going to LIKE IT whether you want to or not." And then she burped and shit her pants. I took that as a sign that all systems were GO.

The family drove up to the trailhead in three separate cars. We would have taken four cars but that seemed *excessive.* The surrounding scenery was indescribably beautiful, a portrait of snowcapped mountains and acres of pine trees dotted intermittently by tiny streams.

And I remember thinking to myself that it was totally worth it; I was so glad we decided to shatter all semblance of Leta's daily schedule and walk a mile up that gorgeous mountain where there was no hot water to make a bottle and no soft surface to take a nap. She was liking it even though she didn't want to like it. I was Master of the Universe.

And that's when God decided to smite me with his sword of Screaming Leta.

With no hot water to make a bottle and no soft surface on which to take a nap, we found ourselves assaulted by an inconsolable force of fury. On the side of a mountain. In the sun. By a lake. With pretty trees.

I tried plying her with beef jerky and all ten of my yummy fingers. I tried walking her up and down the path while singing every song in the Morrissey catalogue. I idiotically tried to feed her a cold bottle with cold milk and a cold nipple and was met with a reaction that said, "You are a wretched fiend-mother. I would rather you offer me a witch's tit."

And that's when the anxiety attack hit, my mouth spewing forbidden obscenities in front of my mother and several innocent nieces and nephews. And I began running back down the mountain clutching Leta to my chest in an effort to shield innocent birds and squirrels and baby rabbits from the screaming sword of God's wrath. Jon followed closely behind carrying all of our gear and speaking rational words of logical logic to guide us down the trail.

About twenty steps into our descent God opened up the heavens and began to rain down upon my wickedness heavy golf-ball-sized hail. I managed to hold Leta close enough that her head was spared any pelting from the golf balls even though she tried every maneuver in her repertoire to pry herself from my grasp, arching her back and pushing her body away from mine. It was like she knew there were golf balls falling from the sky and she was trying to catch them with her mouth.

Rain and hail and wind and screaming followed us the entire hike back down the mountain, and when we got back to the car she continued to scream until we could warm a bottle up in front of the heating vents. We were soaking wet and bruised from God's game of miniature golf.

That was probably the lowest point of the week, other low points being screaming matches between certain members of my family and the throwing of keys BY SOMEONE OTHER THAN ME! And then there was the constant fear that certain nephews might crush Leta's skull by walking back and forth around her play area, except these nephews had never really *walked* anywhere in their lives, unless you could place stomping and thrashing in the same category as a leisurely stroll.

We were so happy to drive home and sleep in our own beds, to dodge flying objects thrown only by me. Leta took two two-hour naps the day we got home as if to say, God thinks you deserve a break, Crazy Lady. No more enclosed quarters with my lovely family who all eat hot dogs with no buns, no more revving ATVs, no more hiking through hostile territory, NO MORE GRUMPY BABY.

At the beginning of August Jon took several days of government-sanctioned Family Leave to watch over me as I tried a new round of hard-core drugs laden with side effects. By this point I had already tried Risperdal, Ativan, Trazodone, Lamictal, Effexor, Abilify, Strattera, Klonopin, and Seroquel. I couldn't sleep, couldn't unclench my jaw or hands, couldn't imagine how I would get through another ten minutes.

I was also terrified of the strain that this was putting on my marriage. Jon was in the middle of a huge project at work, and in order to get time off he risked the wrath of an unforgiving boss. I watched the lines around his eyes multiply when he would come home expecting a hug after a day of being belittled in front of his coworkers only to have me storm out of the house screaming, "IT'S *YOUR* TURN!" Or to discover that I had been so frustrated with the collapsible stroller that I had thrown it off the porch into the yard and then slammed the front door so hard that the doorknob had fallen off. Jon routinely came home to a broken house and a broken wife, and I often felt like I had broken his life.

Taking family leave from his job had been his idea because he was done dealing with my unpredictable outbursts. Every day he brought up the idea that I should check myself into the hospital because he didn't want to go on living this way, why did I? So that's why I agreed to try new drugs, because I could see how I was slowly driving my husband away.

I was already well aware of the terrible things the drugs could do to me and had on occasion read threads on a few message boards where people shouted OH MY GOD THAT DRUG WILL KILL YOU at each other, and in such a fragile state I didn't need strangers predicting my death in all caps. I'd done the research and had rolled out of bed feeling like someone had scraped out my guts and replaced them with a colony of maggots. One of the drugs I tried had the potential to cause a deadly skin rash. A killer rash! That kills people! At the end of one of my therapy sessions I half-jokingly asked the doctor, "Who dies from a skin rash?" as if to say, "Who is such a pussy that they would fall over from a few red bumps?" For the previous hour I had detailed my elaborate state of pussiness, and I wanted him to be able to make a speech at my funeral about how I was able to make jokes about my condition up until the last layer of skin peeled from my body. "She was a funny girl, if not a total pussy," he would say.

The whole thing reminded me of the semester I studied in England my senior year in college. I spent a lot of time with a family in North London, a family with three young kids who could solve the world's energy crisis with the force of their collective brain power. During my first dinner with the family the two-year-old girl explained to me that the vegetables were "delightfully organic as mum prefers it that way." And then she smiled and looked off into the distance as if something had just occurred to her, perhaps the delightful solution to cold fusion.

After dinner the mother took all three kids upstairs to prepare them for their nighttime bath, and soon after the six-year-old son came traipsing downstairs to make faces at me at the bottom of the stairs. He was completely nude except for a dog tag hanging around his neck. His father, who was sitting next to me, motioned the naked boy over so that he could come show me his *penile disease.*

Blink.

Blink. Blink.

I was perfectly comfortable with the fact that the boy was nude as I had read about young boys and their nudeness in philosophy. But I was in no way comfortable or interested in getting a closer look at this young lad's penile disease, and as he skipped closer I scrambled for a way to say to his father, "You know, he probably has a great penile disease and I'm sure you're very proud of it, but can't I just trust you on this one?"

But how do you say that to someone? How do you actually utter the words "penile disease" to a distinguished British father who is obviously very happy to trot out his son's disorder? And so I did what any other American would do in this situation and I screamed, "PENILE DIS-EASE? *PENILE DISEASE??!!*"

Sensing my disbelief his father assured me, "Yes! A penile disease!" And then he informed me further that it was "indeed very nasty and grave." And then he went on to describe how common these penile diseases were among young kids, all while the boy skipped closer and closer with his diseased penile. At this point he was singing a diseased penile ditty with the words, "I've got a penile disease! I've got a penile disease!" while clomping his bare feet to the rhythm, his diseased penile bouncing up and down. I wanted to die, or at least disappear and never again be confronted with the vision of a diseased penile clomping its nudeness toward my defenseless non-peniled self.

And as the walls of the room were about to collapse on my dizzying, frenzied panic, as the air became harder and harder to inhale, the father reached down to his son, lifted up the dog tag, and showed me the inscription: "This child suffers from a peanut allergy."

Peanut.

Allergy.

A peanut disease.

My world did an automatic flip-flop when I realized that we had been speaking two different versions of English and I said, "PEANUT? *PEANUT* DISEASE??" And his father, without missing a beat again assured me, "That's what I said. Penile disease."

I was so relieved that I reached down and hugged the nude non-peanut eater and bellowed, "I LOVE YOUR PEANUT DISEASE!"

And he said back sadly, "I can't eat peniles. They give me a rash."

• • •

During Leta's appointment for her six-month immunizations we had to prepare her for a third round of injections. During her second-month and fourth-month procedures she cried for all of four seconds each time, but that time she bawled open-mouthed, pausing between screams with a silence that made each subsequent scream unbearable, like the eerie silence before a tornado picks up a double-wide and then throws the son of a bitch two miles across town.

Tears puddled underneath her head on the white butcher paper lining the inspection table, and I hugged her arms and held her head in my hands as I let go of my own emotion and cried in rhythm with her tears. Even though I knew that every other child goes through this, I felt like they were picking on Leta and I wanted to punch the nurse in the nose. Wasn't there a more gentle way to deliver the injections, perhaps a pill? Or maybe a blessing in the child's general direction? Whose brilliant idea was it to protect the world from these diseases by JABBING BABIES WITH NEEDLES? Why were we covering light sockets with protective plastic coverings when doctors everywhere were poking infants with sharp, disease-infested objects? Parenthood makes no sense.

Immunizations always messed with Leta's sleeping habits and left her aching all night with a high fever. I'd been worried about this particular round of immunizations because we had worked so hard to get her to sleep through the night, and for almost two months straight she had slept at least eleven to twelve hours every night without waking up. The night of the immunizations, however, she was awake at 2:30, 3:30, 4, 5:30, 6, and finally 6:45 AM bellowing her discomfort in moans and wails and screeches. I knew that she was just a baby and she had no idea what she was doing, but this behavior led me to believe that she had inherited the Hamilton sick gene. This meant that when she was sick the whole world had to suffer with her.

I got confirmation of her Hamilton sick gene when at 2:30 AM she made a horrible, ground-shaking gag noise as I tried to give her Infants' Tylenol. It was a sound I recognized from childhood, a sound that used to echo off the walls in my house and bounce off the inner core of the Earth when my father was perched over a toilet and dry-heaving his empty stomach out his face.

My father never vomited quietly. When he gagged he gagged with his entire body, his whole torso writhing and twitching to the cadence of dead souls coming out of his mouth in booming stereo surround. He would wake up the whole house in the middle of the night because the family wasn't allowed to sleep when he was sick. That wouldn't have been fair. It was the loudest noise of my childhood, louder than any severe thunderstorm or locomotive engine, until my brother hit puberty and assumed the legacy. There was no louder noise in this world than a sixteen-year-old Hamilton pubescent puking SpaghettiOs at 5:30 AM on a Monday morning. When my brother was sick all of Western Tennessee wasn't allowed to sleep.

None of us slept very much that night, which wasn't that big of a deal when you consider the fact that I already had a sleeping disorder and didn't sleep much anyway. While listening to Leta moan I lay awake thinking about how she had peed while lying naked on the scale at the doctor's office—not just a little pee but a gushing fountain of pee, waterfalls of pee, pee that you usually see flowing out of the mouth of a sculpture in the middle of a public town square. I didn't know whether to be embarrassed or to throw in a few pennies and make a wish.

And then I thought about how we had this baby who was half asleep and moaning in the next room, a kid with flesh and blood and hair and a fully functioning excretory system. I had a baby who sometimes looked like me, who sometimes reminded me of my father. I didn't care that it was usually mid-gag while waking up a good portion of the world's Mormon population. Somehow that seemed fair.

CHAPTER FOURTEEN

Heather, Interrupted

*A*fter weeks of threatening to leave Jon if he had me committed to a hospital, I finally gave in and committed myself. I told him that I wanted him to drive me to the hospital and sit with me as I checked into the psychiatric ward. I was afraid that if I didn't go ahead and do it that I would experience some sort of nervous breakdown.

My anxiety had only gotten worse since I started seeing a therapist three months earlier. It was so bad that it choked me every day, and sometimes I couldn't even walk because my body was paralyzed with anxiety. I'd tried over ten different medications and each one had made my anxiety worse. The depression came and went and then came again, but the anxiety was constant. I could barely eat anything and couldn't sleep, even though I'd tried every sleeping pill available at the pharmacy. I wanted to commit suicide if only because then I wouldn't have to feel the pain of being awake anymore.

I couldn't believe that I didn't feel better. I couldn't believe that it had been three months and I DIDN'T FEEL ANY BETTER.

I had to believe that going to the hospital would at least let me clear my head, or that it might actually provide an answer. I had to believe in something because I didn't feel like I had any hope. The anxiety was so painful, and I couldn't see an end to it.

Six months after having all my instincts turn on and go haywire I still couldn't turn them off, or even turn them down. Those instincts turned into demons that terrorized me from the moment I got out of bed in the morning to the hours and hours that I tried to sleep at night. I never had a moment of peace.

I just didn't feel better.

When I checked myself in to the hospital I felt like a crazed kid at a concert who had, in a moment of sheer insanity, jumped off the stage in a grand, sweeping swan dive.

The first night there was probably the worst night of my life. They didn't have any beds in the unlocked unit of the facility so they stuck me in the least scary locked unit, the one whose occupants averaged over eighty-two years in age. Everything smelled of urine, including the plastic eating utensils. Everyone referred to me as "kiddo" and that was very cute and endearing and all, but I was LOCKED INSIDE A MENTAL INSTITUTION.

The views out the windows of the facility were oddly beautiful. The building sat at the curve of a small hill overlooking the entire Salt Lake Valley. In one direction I could see sweeping hills and nooks and canyons dotted with green desert plants that looked like dusty velvet.

In the other direction I saw an open field of lights and streets that seemed to extend for hundreds of miles, and it felt like I was hovering over the whole scene. I could see the Mormon temple from up there, or at least the buildings in downtown that surround and protect it. I imagine that Brigham Young was standing in a place similar to this one when he looked over the valley and decided that "this was the place" to settle the Mormons. By saying that I am in no way implying that he was a crazed lunatic. Not at all. Nope.

Inside the facility, however, the lights were fluorescent and the food was plastic. Some of the food even JIGGLED. When I arrived on a Thursday afternoon I was in such a bad place that I couldn't sit still to read a magazine, and the fluorescent glow in my room was flickering like a sequence in a horror film. All I could do was curl up in my bed and pull the covers over my head. I couldn't believe I was there.

I had given my story to at least three different people—an intake social worker, a nurse, and a doctor—so I thought that they understood that I had a severe and unbearable case of insomnia. I remember saying out loud three different times: "I DON'T SLEEP. EVER." That night as I prepared to go to bed I asked someone at the front desk if they could give me something to sleep, and the guy on duty plopped down a pill that I had tried before, a pill that hadn't ever worked.

So I said, "This pill doesn't work."

And he said, "This is the only thing I am allowed to give you."

Four hours later after trying and trying to go to sleep I wandered back out to the front desk and asked for something else, PLEASE GIVE ME SOMETHING ELSE. There was a new girl at the desk and she checked my chart and informed me, "It says here that I'm not allowed to give you anything else. Sorry."

WHAT KIND OF THERAPY WAS THIS?

So I didn't sleep that night. Not a wink. And every time the girl from the front desk came to check on me—every fifteen minutes, with a flashlight, in my face, because I'm a CRAZIE!—I would sit up straight in bed and say, "HI! I'm STILL AWAKE!" By morning she was checking on me from the hallway and saying back, "Hi! You're still awake. I get it."

Friday morning I finally saw my official doctor, an amazing psychiatrist who had been treating people like me for longer than I had been alive. He had read my chart—imagine that! He had done some research! On me! His patient! And within the first five minutes of talking to me he determined why and how the meds I'd been taking weren't working. He had such a direct approach, almost like a bulldozer with a PhD, and I wanted to smother him with love. I could tell that he wanted to see me get better and knowing that he cared, even just a little bit, made me feel SO MUCH BETTER.

I did my best to impress him, to make him believe that underneath the Crazie was a solid individual because I so desperately wanted to be unlocked. By the end of our session he had ordered me a transfer to the unlocked unit, a place where I could come and go without being followed by someone with a flashlight.

Because I was under constant supervision, I was able to take therapeutic quantities of drugs immediately: 40mg of Prozac, 10mg of Valium, 2400mg of Neurontin. That amount of Neurontin could probably knock out an entire herd of buffalo, but because my anxiety was so bad, it did nothing but enable me to sit still. For the first time since Leta was born. It was a combination he had given to countless women who had suffered postpartum depression, one that had worked time and time again. I felt a difference within two hours, and if you ask Jon he will tell you that when he saw me that afternoon he saw Heather for the first time in seven months, not that awful woman who liked to throw keys at his head. I truly believe that my doctor in the hospital saved my life. *I owe that man my life.*

And everything in the unlocked unit was more tolerable. I would have even called some things wonderful. I took a nap that afternoon—a nap with dreams and slobbering drool on my pillow—and that was a sign of healing if there ever was one. A nap!

My new meds seemed to be working in the sense that I hadn't had any horrifying side effects, and I was able to sit down and read two whole *Us Weekly* magazines. TWO! I knew more about the cast of *The O.C.* than I EVER WANTED TO KNOW.

Jon visited me at least twice a day and we had several meals together. One afternoon he brought a runny-nosed and grumpy Leta to lunch and we fed her mushed croutons and refried beans. Sadly, Jon had to change the refried bean diaper the next morning. I think he may have described it as UNPLEASANT.

Jon was a Superhero throughout the whole thing, and I was once again reminded that I scored the Best Husband in All the Land. He was so supportive and giving and so very, very hot. I missed him so much that I physically hurt, and when he visited I plunged my face into his neck so that I could smell the shaving cream he had used earlier in the day. That was my favorite smell in the world, right up there with the smell of Leta's head and the smell of bacon frying.

When my friends and family said that they couldn't believe I was being so open about this, I wanted to ask them WHY NOT? Why should there be any shame in getting help for a disease?

If there is a stigma to this, let there be one. At least I was alive. At least my baby still had her mother. At least I had a chance at a better life.

Being in the hospital was strange if not incredibly boring. There were only two televisions for a group of over thirty people and the channel was always turned to the Olympics. I had nothing against the Olympics; in fact I found the little platform divers very cute in their little

Speedos, and I loved it when they flipped off those precipices and made cute little splashes with their cute little selves. I found myself wanting to pinch their little butts and to feed them a warm bottle.

The only problem I had with the TV being permanently tuned to the Olympics was the Bob Costas factor. Please, Bob Costas, JUST SHUT UP. Why did he have to scar this precious world with his insipid voice-over? How many potentially wonderful and touching moments had been ruined by his droning commentary? It wasn't healthy for me to carry around so much hate, but I'd been watching Bob Costas for FOUR STRAIGHT DAYS. In the loony bin. There was no better place to carry around hate than in the hospital because they were monitoring me. I couldn't throw things in there.

Other than hating Bob Costas I read magazines, listened to PJ Harvey, and talked to the other Crazies. I couldn't help talking to the other Crazies because they cornered me and FORCED ME TO LISTEN. One morning some stranger trapped me and gave me his life story for over an hour. I was being nice and listening closely up until the thirty-minute mark when I realized that he was repeating himself, and for the next thirty minutes I heard the whole story of his life for the fifth and sixth time. I knew as much about that stranger as I did the cast of *The O.C.* My brain was verging on explosion.

I had an incredible roommate who was sent home the day before I was, a charming twenty-year-old girl. She was starting her first year at BYU that week, and she was the spitting image of one of the roommates I had had at BYU. When I was talking to her I was reminded of some of the great times I had as a college student, times spent being creative in such an oppressive environment. My roommates and I used to drive up to 7-Eleven in the middle of the night and fill up 64-ounce

Diet Dr Peppers. We'd spend the rest of the night and morning giggling while on a caffeine and saccharine high talking about the guys we'd really like to make out with. Of course, all making out would be in a vertical position, fully clothed, with no roaming hands and touching of the sacred parts.

I knew I was getting better because not once did I try to convince her that she should run as far as she could from BYU. In fact, I told her that she'd have a blast, and I wished her all the luck in the world. DEAR LORD, WHAT HAD I BECOME? There was sunshine in my soul! I could stop exclamation pointing!

I saw my doctor one final time for a follow-up assessment, and we talked about how common my condition is among women whose bodies are transforming from a pregnant being to a non-pregnant being, and he told me about all the chemical and hormonal things that can go wrong. He had treated hundreds of women just like me, women who had gone on to have multiple children without any relapse of depression, and I felt very encouraged. He assured me that what I was feeling was easily treatable, and he was certain that the new meds I was on would kick my anxiety and pain in the butt.

I cannot express how much I liked this doctor. I felt a huge sense of relief and safety in being under the care of someone who knew so much about how to treat postpartum depression. At one point in our conversation he set down his pen and paper, paused, and then looked at me and said, "You poor woman. I am so sorry for what you have been through." And I cried. I cried hard. My God, what I had been through.

I know that people had experienced far worse pain than I had, far worse trials and lots in life. But my pain was real, and to me it had been unbearable and incapacitating. It had also affected my family, and for that reason alone I had to get help.

I was discharged only four days after I had checked in, and it wasn't a moment too soon. I'd missed my family. I'd missed my dog. I'd missed my daily Pop-Tart.

I felt good about going home. I felt like there was an open road in front of me, a road to joy and happiness. I felt like I had a new perspective on things. That was what the hospital stay had provided me: PERSPECTIVE. It had also provided me an appreciation for my regular toothpaste and deodorant. The first time I brushed my teeth with the hospital toothpaste I gagged and was certain I had grabbed a tube of ointment instead of toothpaste, perhaps the kind you might apply to an open wound or a swollen anus; it couldn't have been safe for my mouth. And the deodorant! They gave me deodorant that smelled like the shavings that line the bottom of a gerbil cage. I SMELLED LIKE A GERBIL.

Dear Leta,

Today you turn seven months old. Some people might say that there is nothing special about turning seven months old; you can't get your driver's license or purchase alcohol in a manner that wouldn't get you arrested. But what they don't know is that with the seven-month mark comes the POP-TART AND PICKLES PRIVILEGE. What could be more special than that?

Just this morning your father and I spent over a half hour sharing our strawberry Pop-Tart with you, giving you little bites with the yummy strawberry filling. You gummed the pieces with sheer delight, making mmmm, mmmm noises and waving your hands like some beauty pageant winner on a float being pulled down Main Street. Several times you tried to grab the Pop-Tart out of my hand, but OH, NO, little Scooter. I didn't want strawberry Pop-Tart all over the walls or stuck in my hair or flung through the window into the driveway. You've got quite an arm on you. You could break land-speed records with the toys you throw.

I know that the Pop-Tart police are going to contact me and accuse me of feeding you something that will turn you into a homicidal sociopath later in life, because that's what Pop-Tarts do, they corrupt and demoralize and subvert Heavenly Father's plan, but oh how I'll love my cute little homicidal sociopath.

A couple of days ago we put you in the high chair and fed you Cheerios. Oh Mary Mother of God how you love those crunchy, oaty O's. I think it may be an instinct kicking in, your love of Cheerios. There must have been a primitive form of Cheerios in prehistoric times, because I don't know how the species could have prospered if Cro-Magnon babies didn't have their Cheerios. What would they throw across the room or drop off their high chairs to feed Cro-Magnon puppies?

You're barely big enough to see over the tray in the high chair, but you're pretty good at reaching your hands up and grabbing handfuls of Cheerios. Gobs and gobs you grab, and you bring a fistful of O's to your mouth, but that's where you become stumped, like, I've got them close to my mouth, NOW WHAT DO I DO? Some of them make it to your chin, others to your ears, but most of them end up on the floor and in Chuck's mouth. That was Happy Hour for Chuck, billions and billions of treats on the floor. He snarfed so many Cheerios that the house smelled of oaty dog farts for the rest of the day.

Your relationship with Chuck is remarkable. He loves to lick your face after you've been fed a bottle, and you sit there with your nose scrunched up and your eyes closed in a state of half bliss and half wonder. Who is this beast that lives in your house? This beast with fur and fangs and wiry whiskers that tickle when he sniffs your face? Whenever he enters the room you stare at him in amazement and then giggle for no reason other than the fact that this creature exists. Chuck is happy to amuse you, you who have come into this house and disrupted his peaceful life as the only child, you who consume most of Mama's attention, but I think he's devising certain plans that involve lifting his leg and peeing on whomever you bring home as your first date. That will be his way of saying, WHO'S GIGGLING NOW?

A few days ago I came home from the hospital after getting help for my disease. I happened to come home just as you were waking up from your first morning nap, and when I walked into your room your smell hit me like a monsoon. That was one of the most peaceful moments of my life, being wrapped with the blanket of your fragrance, knowing that I would get to spend the whole day with you. When I picked you up out of the crib you looked at me and smiled, your trademark gummy smile, and this look of recognition flashed across your face that said, "You are the woman who used to feed me with your boobs, and now you are that woman who snorts and tries to make me laugh, and you eat my feet a lot. I remember you! Hey! It's YOU!"

Leta, I need you to understand that I went to the hospital because something was wrong inside of me. My disease is not your fault, and you are not the reason that I am sick. When you are old enough to read and understand these things I don't want you to blame yourself for the pain I have been through. Nor do I want you to be ashamed that your mother had to go to the hospital. I am not ashamed. In fact, I couldn't be happier about the help that I received. I feel better, and I haven't been able to say that in such a long time.

I think you have noticed a difference in me because you have been utterly joyous these past few days. You are constantly smiling and giggling, laughing out loud with your whole body. And the noises that come out of your mouth span the whole alphabet. Your father and I just sit and stare at you, amazed that such an extraordinary being sprouted from the two of us. In case anyone hasn't told you yet, you look a lot like your father. You look a lot like his father, actually, and sometimes we call you Byron Junior. When your father brought you into the hospital to see me, the staff at the front desk would say, "Oh how sweet, he looks just like his father."

You are my sweet Zing Zing Zing Bah, my Punkin Head Piggy. I love you, and I missed you like crazy. It's great to be home.

Love, Mama

Her Screamness Who Screams a Lot
Every Day With the Screaming

*I*t's impossible to describe how hard it is to take care of an infant day in and day out without a break on the weekends. It's just not something you can understand unless you've actually experienced it, and I like to refer to parenthood as "being on the other side." It's like I crossed over some invisible line, and once I did the whole world changed. Now when friends of mine have their first child I usually say to them, "Welcome to the other side. It only gets worse from here."

That sounds pessimistic, I know, and of course there are many wonderful things about having a baby. But when we had Leta on that cold February morning it was like a bomb exploded in our house, and we were slowly putting the pieces back together. One night in early September Jon and I were trying to figure out how we'd made it this far. How did we make it through sleepless night after sleepless night, and the screaming? THE INCESSANT, NEVER-ENDING, SKIN-MELTING SCREAMING! I don't know how anyone could make it through this battlefield without going crazy.

I went crazy. Somewhere along the road of putting everything back together I broke down. But going to the hospital was the best decision I had made as a mother. And I made that decision as a mother with the health of my child as my singular goal. Making that decision was as instinctual as feeding her and clothing her. I felt so much better and was sleeping through the night. Hours and hours and hours of sleeping! And when I woke up in the morning my immediate thought was BRING IT ON. Whatever the child threw at me—hours of cranky bleating, diapers with nuggets of noxious, rotting nuclear fallout, short naps and subsequent tired groaning—I could take it.

I could take it!

In the weeks following my hospital stay Leta and I formed a bond that was unable to take form when I was in my anxious, clenched state of unhappiness. She responded to the new look in my face, the look that said, "I am winning this war." She was constantly giggling and cooing and slurping and kicking her frog feet in glee. And I just couldn't get enough of her.

Because of this new bond I had a difficult time one afternoon when the new babysitter we hired came to take care of her for a few hours. As part of my ongoing therapy we hired someone to come help with the care of Leta for nine hours a week while I worked on writing and free-lance projects. It was just nine hours, per week. That was fewer hours than *The Lord of the Rings* trilogy. That was fewer hours than the sleep I got in one night. BUT OH THE GUILT THAT SHOOK ME TO THE CORE.

I sat in the basement trying to work, but I wanted to throw up the entire time. How could I leave my baby in the care of someone who would play with her and feed her a bottle? How wicked and uncaring of a mother could I be? I might as well throw her in the middle of the street and walk away, OH LOATHSOME EXCUSE OF A PARENT!

Not once did she cry; in fact, I could hear her laughing and having a good time upstairs. But downstairs my soul withered as unbearable guilt took hold of my being and twisted it like a dirty wet rag. So I tried to work, and then I cleaned the entire basement, dusting the crevices with a Q-tip to keep my mind off the fact that I had abandoned my baby upstairs with a caring, qualified babysitter.

My friends had told me that this would get easier with time, that the guilt would fade because HEY! LOOK! Other mothers had gone back to work after having a baby! And the world still turned! But that first afternoon with the new babysitter my world stopped, and God, I missed her.

And you know what? Sometimes it's *okay* to miss your kids. I was learning to be okay.

When Leta was diagnosed with torticollis plagiocephaly at two months old, a condition defined by the way she tilted her her head in a certain direction that caused her head to grow in a misshapen form, we began months of rigorous physical therapy with her and cured the torticollis (titling of the head) and the shape of her head filled out nicely into the round shape of a normal human skull. But when she got really tired or slightly sick she resorted to tilting her head again. This really worried me and so I took her back to the physical therapist for a re-assessment.

After several exercises and an hour of observation her physical therapist assured me that Leta's neck was perfectly okay, but that I should be much more worried about the fact that she refused to put any weight whatsoever on her legs. She determined that Leta hated the sensation of pressure on her feet, like someone might hate the sound of fingernails being scraped down a chalkboard. She gave me a list of exercises that I had to put Leta through every day to get her used to pressure on her feet, and OH MY GOD SHE HATED IT.

After every diaper change I picked her up, held her firmly against me with one arm, and with my other arm I forced her legs to become straight underneath her. Then I leaned forward and placed all of her weight on her legs. And she screamed. Like I was cutting her with a knife. And then she screamed more, like MAMA PLEASE STOP YOU'RE KILLING ME. I tried not to cry.

In the middle of playtime with the elephant that rattles and the soft yellow duck that quacks I'd straddle her on my leg and force her legs to stiffen on the floor. And she screamed. Why did I have to disrupt play-time with the elephant and the duck? The elephant and the duck were so much nicer than Mama, she who forced the chubby little feet to meet the floor. The chubby little feet hated the floor, oh hard and flat surface! The floor was hard! And flat! And extended in all directions! There was no escape!

After a few weeks of these new exercises we didn't see much improve-ment, so her pediatrician suggested that we get an MRI done on her head to make sure everything was in working order. He told me that he wanted to calm my fears that anything might be wrong because he was certain that Leta was perfectly healthy. But ordering an MRI for a child of someone in my postpartum, anxious condition was like throwing someone who can't swim into a lake to assure them that not being able to swim is perfectly okay. And even though my meds were working I was nervous simply about the fact that I had to take my child *to a hospital for a procedure.*

My mother, the Avon World Sales Leader, postponed her weekly trip to LA to be with us, and Jon took an entire day off work to give me support. Leta awoke that morning to her usual bottle, or so she thought as she grabbed it in hunger. We couldn't feed her anything but clear liquids in the hours leading up to the MRI, which I was already skeptical about considering she'd been fed nothing but non-clear liquid every single day of her life. She hadn't taken a bottle since 6 PM the previous night, and so she was starving like a normal baby who hadn't had anything to eat in thirteen hours. You'd think that the taste of something delightfully fruity! and sweet! and did I mention fruity! would sit well on the palate of an infant who gobbled applesauce and Twizzlers like a starved monkey at the zoo who is just so damn cute that you can't obey the sign that says DO NOT FEED MONKEYS TWIZZLERS. But this infant was the offspring of an Armstrong and a Hamilton, and that meant her sole purpose in life was to make everything difficult for everyone else. There should be a law against two people from Scottish lineage mating and releasing monsters into the world.

We spent the entire morning distracting her from the fact that she was hungry, and we did this by giving her things that she could shove into her mouth: measuring cups, spoons, sharp knives, and matches. HAHA! Just kidding about the matches. It's amazing what the art of distraction can do to a grumpy infant. If her mood had been traced by a monitor that morning it would have looked like a series of mountains and valleys, the valleys being the two seconds that she realized OH MY GOD I'M HUNGRY, and the mountains being the next sixty seconds of Jon making a silly face or me finding an object in the house that she hadn't ever seen and shoving it in her hands. By the time we had to leave for the hospital we were at a point where we were about to take apart the computers to show her what a motherboard looks like. THERE JUST WEREN'T ANY MORE OPTIONS.

We'd been to this particular hospital before and were prepared for the harrowing experience it is to see children in various states of pain and disease. Still, nothing can really protect your heart from witnessing children in wheelchairs or children with tubes in their ears and noses, and I tried to concentrate on the fact that this MRI was a preventative measure, not something she had to undergo because of a diagnosed disease. As I was walked through the halls I had never been more thankful for my health, for my husband's health, and for the screaming, whiny, grumpy health of my cranky Leta Elise.

After we checked in and Leta had her vitals taken we were told that we would have to keep her awake for another forty-five minutes before they could give her the sedative, something called Nembutal that would be delivered orally and not intravenously THANK THE LORD GOD OF EVERY RELIGION ON EARTH. However, it was already over an hour past Leta's nap time, and we were going to have to keep her awake for another forty-five minutes? Did they not have any idea who they were dealing with? Had they not heard of Her Screamness Who Screams a Lot Every Day With the Screaming? I started to panic a little bit, and Jon, sensing my discomfort and afraid I might make a scene, haunted by the echoes of my unpredictable outbursts, whisked Leta away to be with the Avon World Sales Leader in the waiting room. When he came back to me he assured me that everything was okay, and COME ON! If anyone can keep that baby awake it's That Woman With All The Jewelry.

Of course, the Avon World Sales Leader did not disappoint, and while keeping Leta awake without any screaming she also made a 40 percent sales increase for the Western Region of Avon *she was that good.* Plus, she had on a festive, patriotic scarf. I would have stayed awake for her, too.

When it came time to sedate Leta, I held her down on the table while a nurse shot a hefty portion of Nembutal into Leta's gagging, very cute mouth. Leta didn't cry, she just made that loud Hamilton gagging sound, like the sound of a sick hippopotamus wailing in the mud. The nurse told me that I could hold her as the sedative took effect, and so I tried to cuddle Leta to my shoulder as she went under. What happened next will go down as one of the funniest eight-minute periods of my life. My baby was drunk. Not just drunk but D.R.U.N.K. She was as drunk as a sixteen-year-old on prom night who has had a Long Island Iced Tea on an empty stomach and is in total denial about how drunk she is.

For eight minutes my child tried to deny her state of drunkenness, and she giggled and laughed and blew raspberries and bobbed her head about four hundred times. If she had been able to talk she would have said, "I pomnise nat I am dot nrunk. No, I neam it! I'm dot nrunk!" And she fought it and fought it. I've never seen her giggle so much, and I'm just glad that she was immobile and not staggering into walls or falling over on other people LIKE HER MOTHER DOES WHEN SHE IS DOT NRUNK.

After eight hilarious, head-bobbing minutes she finally passed out on my shoulder, as still as a pitch black night. She went very limp and became very heavy, and since I had been warned about this I wasn't too upset when I felt her that way in my arms. We laid her down on the table and waited for the call to be taken into the MRI room. I think for both Jon and myself it was a treat to see Leta so asleep, her eyes closed and her body so still. Leta had always put herself to sleep, so we rarely got a glimpse of her when she was in this state, and when we did the room was dark and we were trying not to wake her up. She looked so helpless, so tiny and fragile. So little. In those few moments before the MRI we got to be with our sleeping little Leta, and HOLY SHIT! We made a baby! I had never felt so startled at that realization.

When the nurse strapped her onto the MRI table I almost lost my breakfast on the floor, and that was the moment when the mama bear inside of me roared and wanted to claw out the eyes of everyone in the room. She lay there strapped into this contraption, so lifeless and still, and I couldn't do anything at that point. I had to stand by and watch that part happen and I'd never felt so helpless. The MRI room was straight out of a scene in *Willy Wonka,* a gigantic thing-a-magoogy sitting in the middle with all these Disney stickers slapped on its side. There were Disney stickers all over the walls there to distract children from the fact that they were being STRAPPED AGAINST THEIR WILL INTO A MACHINE THAT WOULD SUCK OUT THEIR BRAIN! RUN! RUN! I expected Gene Wilder to hop out of the thing-a-magoogy and say, "Is the grisly reaper mowing? Yes, the danger must be growing, 'cause the rowers keep on rowing, and they're certainly not showing, any signs that they are slowing!"

OH MY GOD I ALMOST FREAKED OUT! AND IT WAS LOUD! MY GOD THE NOISE! GENE WILDER! IN PURPLE PANTS!

And then it was over.

Done.

No laser beams or death rays or Oompa-Loompas. The nurse had said that Leta would most likely be asleep for another hour and a half, but we already discovered that the nurses didn't know who was lying there on that machine, and the moment Leta was pulled out of the tunnel she shot awake. And she was not happy, no, not at all, not one bit, and thus commenced Screams a Lot Every Day With the Screaming. I'm not good with hangovers, either, so I would have screamed, too.

She continued screaming in the recovery room, where she drank a bottle of apple juice and two bottles of milk. All of her vitals seemed normal, and after forty-five minutes of Leta's cranky whimpering and screaming the doctor finally came in to give us the good news, that her brain was developing normally, that her skull looked fine, that nothing looked bad. He urged us to keep a close watch on the size of her head in the next few months and warned us that we might want to do another MRI when she turned a year old, just to be safe. There were no words to describe the feeling I had at that news. It felt like the calm as a thunderstorm parts and the sun shoots through the opening in the clouds, and the wind blows the scent of wet leaves and grass into the shadows across the pavement: the feeling of being spared.

The following day she was back to normal, eating Cheerios and stuffing them into her pants. I was suddenly finding Cheerios everywhere, even in the sheets on our bed. She was in a great mood all day and probably had no recollection of being strapped into the Wonkanator, or of being punch drunk and loopy. However, I will always remember those few hours, and the days of worry leading up to those few hours, and the years and years leading up to those days when I didn't know what it was like to have my soul wrapped inside the palm of a baby.

CHAPTER SIXTEEN

If Your Wife Is Pregnant, You Might Want to Skip This One

There is not much that I won't talk about or discuss in great detail with perfect strangers, no topic of conversation off-limits. That is, until I went seven months without having sex.

Seven months after Leta's birth a certain procedure reconvened in the Armstrong household. This procedure was actually the type of procedure that got us into the situation that made reconvening the procedure so difficult, if you know what I'm saying. If you don't know what I'm saying then I'll break this down for you into specifics: when Leta came out of my body she ripped me apart, and the mess that she left—a mess that I felt every stitch of because the epidural had worn off by that point—didn't heal for a very long, long time. So long, in fact, that both my best friend and my sister said to me in the subsequent months, "What? You mean you haven't *done the procedure* yet? Are you serious?"

I AM SERIOUS. And I couldn't find anyone anywhere to back me up. WHERE ARE YOU, PROCEDURE-LESS PERSON?

Some books said that it might take a few weeks (HA!) or months before the procedure could be reconvened, and if you're one of those women who after only six weeks of shoving her boobs down a bottomless opossum could reconvene the procedure with a smile or maybe even an "ooh, yes" then I heartily salute your robotic, adjustable vagina. I bet yours is the type of vagina that can hum show tunes or fold sheets all by itself.

In the middle of all my depression and anxiety and daydreaming about life ending so that the pain might just go away, I honestly thought that I might not ever reconvene the procedure again. By having this baby I had destroyed the procedure part of my life. My doctor assured me that everything had healed the way it should have healed, but that maybe my scar tissue was just tender and that I needed to give it more time.

HOW MUCH TIME IS ENOUGH TIME? I hope this story SCARES THE LIVING SHIT out of some guy out there whose wife is in her third trimester. Ask yourself, buddy, just how long can YOU go without the procedure?

For some women I talked to, three months was the magic number. Others waited four or five months, and I only heard of one other story where they had to wait six whole months to reconvene the procedure. Well, this is my story: my vagina can't fold sheets. In fact, my vagina is so retarded that we had to wait to reconvene the procedure until after I had started my period for the first time, after I could stretch it out with A FUCKING TAMPON to get it stabilized for the procedure. YOU CAN'T MAKE THIS SHIT UP.

Jon wrote a Thank You Letter to Tampax, and after the procedure had been reconvened I was so giddy and elated that I wanted to run up and down our street naked shouting to the neighbors, "THE PROCE-

DURE! IT'S BEEN RECONVENED! WAKE UP EVERYBODY!
RECONVENE YOUR PROCEDURE!"

On top of everything that my body had been through with the pregnancy and birth and aftermath, I was unable to reconvene the procedure for seven months and twelve days. And on each and every one of
those days I had the thought that I might not ever be able to reconvene
the procedure. I had friends with children Leta's age, friends who were
already pregnant again, three and four and five months pregnant, meaning their procedures reconvened in a timely, penis-friendly fashion.
Where did these people get their vaginas? Did they trade in their
brains?

I want to end this story with just one other tiny detail, the part about
how I got a urinary tract infection *from reconvening the procedure.* I
woke up a few days after the incident peeing fire and blood into the
toilet, unable to veer more than a few feet from the bathroom the entire
day. I wanted to laugh about this, because this was ridiculous, and
THEY DON'T TELL YOU ABOUT THIS STUFF when you take
your baby home from the hospital, that in seven months when your
vagina finally heals and you're able to reconvene your procedure, there
will be one day when your baby will spend her entire day in the high
chair next to the toilet.

The Mormon Church holds a general assembly meeting twice a year, a
meeting called General Conference where the leaders of the Church
give talks about the same stuff you have to hear about over and over
again in Sunday school every Sunday, stuff like: 1) The importance of
being faithful, 2) The importance of prayer in our lives, 3) The impor-

tance of serving others, 4) The importance of reading the scriptures, 5) The importance of tithing, and 6) The importance of thong panties.

General Conference is always the most boring meeting in the history of religion on earth. They always give the same talks about the same things and there is always one story about how someone learned an important lesson while attending to the cows on the farm he grew up on in Idaho. And at one point someone will say a sentence that involves the word MOUNTAIN and it will come out sounding like MAO-IN, because that's how they say things in Utah, and I will take a steak knife and gouge out my eye.

Not that I would be watching.

In Utah the Mormons can just roll out of bed and watch Conference because the local NBC affiliate is owned by the Mormon Church and hey! There's the Prophet on Channel 5! In Utah, General Conference is like a vacation from having to go to church because you can sit there nude and watch all the talks while eating Cheetos. But in other places, places far away like Tennessee where I grew up, the Mormons actually have to get dressed up and go to church and watch it via satellite. And they have to sit there and try not to fall asleep or become suffocated because the panty hose their mothers made them wear is cutting off circulation to the lower halves of their bodies.

We sent Leta to Conference Camp one weekend in October so that my mother could watch her for two days while Jon and I took the mini-honeymoon we never had up in Park City. It happened to be the same weekend as General Conference, and for two days Leta had to fold her arms and be reverent while the Prophet and the Apostles of the Mormon Church gave talks about thong panties. And while she learned about the importance of prayer and scriptures and tithing and sin and trials and tribulations, Jon and I were sipping bourbon in a hot tub on the deck of a private suite overlooking one of the most beautiful ski resorts in the world.

We arrived at Deer Valley Lodge on a Friday night when the air was crisp and the "deng deng deng deng" guitar riff on every song of an Interpol album was ringing in our ears from having blasted it the entire way. We stood at the check-in desk, drunk on pretzels and Pringles, only to find out that the modest room we had reserved had been mysteriously downgraded to a less than modest room, one without the hot tub. EGAD.

Perhaps it was the pretzels, perhaps it was just the thought of a weekend away from infant management, but neither Jon nor I made a huge fuss; we stood there patiently waiting for the guy at the desk to figure out what went wrong. He apologized for the misunderstanding and I said, "No problem, I used to work for Delta Air Lines and people are crazy. I am not one of those people, so you can take your time." He sighed, relaxed a bit, and said, "I wish every customer were like you." And then he upgraded us to the master suite, a series of rooms bigger than our house with a kitchen and bathroom decked out with granite countertops and travertine tiles. And there was a hot tub, for skinny-dipping.

Being nice! Its pays off! You heard it here first.

We spent the weekend driving through the mountains and hiking in the rain and sleeping for hours and hours in the midafternoon. My God, the sleeping. Jon took a nap with me, for hours. Jon doesn't ever take a nap, and there he was lying next to me, still and lovely and irresistible. We indulged in room service and then got sushi and then ordered champagne at 1 PM in the afternoon for brunch. We ran naked to the hot tub and sat in front of the fireplace to dry off. And then the fire alarm went off.

There's a whole story about the fire alarm and the entire suite being filled with smoke, and I would totally tell it to you but all you need to know is that there was this one moment when I turned to Jon and said, "I'm a little worried about ALL THAT SMOKE POURING OUT OF THE FIREPLACE." And he was all, it's the wood! The wood is green and very smoky! And then the fire alarm went off and the phone rang and the hotel management was all, "MR. ARMSTRONG!"

I can only imagine what the hotel management was thinking, like, that couple is smoking some serious pot for the fucking fire alarm to go off. But the entire suite was filled with smoke, and these guys ran in to figure out what was going on, and I was hiding in the bathroom naked, and they found out that the flue in the fireplace had been shut the entire time. For the rest of the weekend I would turn to Jon and casually say, "It was the wood. The wood was green."

The only other incident worth mentioning was the little bathroom break we took on a hiking trail after driving for an hour in the mountains. Both of our bladders were about to pop, and there were no bathroom facilities within a thirty-mile radius. The trail was clearly marked with a sign that read, "This area is a protected watershed. No animals allowed." Which meant, you are not allowed to use the bathroom here, you Imbecile.

But who was going to know? I had to go pee, and so Jon and I hiked several yards up the trail to a place we thought was out of the way where no one would notice. So I squatted down in the midst of some bushes and trees, and Jon stood nearby because men can do that, just stand there and go pee whereas I HAD TO SQUAT. EMPHASIS COM-

PLETELY JUSTIFIED. And I was going pee, my bare white ass hanging out in nature, and in the middle of my stream a BOY AND HIS FATHER WALKED BY. And when I say walk by, I mean that they passed within THREE FEET of my bare white ass. Jon heard someone talking, and he thought it was me, so he said, "What's up?"

WHAT'S UP?? WHAT'S UP?? HEY BOY AND YOUR FATHER: THERE'S MY WIFE'S BARE WHITE ASS.

I was caught up in the moment of the peeing, and the only thing I could think to do was squat down farther, my bare white ass now touching the forest floor. Oh my God, I had just shown some boy and his father my ass. In the woods. Where I'd been forbidden to pee.

After they passed by I stood up to pull up my pants only to discover that my bare white ass was covered in pine needles. So Jon and I spent the next five minutes picking pine needles out of my panties. I want those five minutes back.

I eventually overcame the embarrassing horror of that moment to enjoy the rest of Our Weekend Away and spent Sunday morning in bed sleeping and sleeping some more until Jon had to push my body out of bed. My reasoning was that I might not ever get to sleep that much again. After we checked out and ate a year's worth of chocolate at the brunch buffet, we headed back out of the mountains, Interpol in the CD player, all of our clothes smelling like smoke from the wood that was green.

One early Wednesday morning I stuck Leta in the BabyBjörn, put the dog on a leash, and took a walk with a friend to a local coffee shop. Leta was dressed entirely in clothes that had been given to her from other people: a shirt from the neighbor, a pair of cut-off denim pants from my mother, and girly socks from Jon's sister. The dog was nude, but he's always nude, so no one really noticed.

I tried to take a walk every day with the wee one and Chuck because Leta had finally learned to love the outdoors, and Chuck loved to sniff vertical objects. It also broke up the monotony of our day. On our walks I usually played with Leta's dangling feet because, well, her feet were dangling, and I was nervous by nature and always looking to fidget with something. Dangling baby feet were perfect for wandering, fidgety hands. And for eating. With ketchup.

On this particular walk, however, I was pretty focused on the conversation I was having with my friend, and I was talking with my hands. I find it physically impossible to utter a single word without waving my hands around in circles like a flight attendant or a castaway trying to flag down a rescue plane. So Leta's feet dangled untouched for pretty much the whole walk while my eyebrows and fingers shouted sentences into the air. When we arrived at the coffee shop I stood outside the door with Chuck on the leash waiting for my friend to get her coffee. I would have bought a coffee as well, but I'd recently figured out that caffeine had no effect on me whatsoever given the whopping amount of a drug that I was on. The drug made me tired, and nothing would deter it. Not even a venti Mocha Valencia with cocaine sprinkled on top.

While I was standing there patiently with the dog on the leash, who by the way was going nuts because there was another dog there sitting reverently next to its owner and Chuck had not yet been given the opportunity to sniff its ass, a woman sitting at one of the outdoor tables turned to the man sitting next to her and whispered, "That baby has only one sock on." I was the only one standing there with a baby attached to my body, and in slow motion I reached down to check Leta's feet and here's where the music from *Psycho* kicked in, when the woman is in the shower and the guy with the knife comes to kill her:

OH. MY. GOD. LETA HAS ONLY ONE SOCK ON. WE HAVE LOST A SOCK. MY BABY IS HALF-SOCKLESS.

There is only one thing in this world that is worse than a sockless baby, and that is a half-sockless baby. When a baby is sockless both of her feet match, so the hobo factor is only moderately high. A half-sockless baby DOES NOT HAVE MATCHING FEET, so the hobo factor is pegged in the red zone, the danger zone, the zone at which the hobo engine is going to overheat and explode.

My first thought was, my husband is going to kill me. My second thought was, Jesus Christ, dog, go sniff that other dog's butt and calm down so that I can freak out. When my friend came out of the coffee shop she saw the look of horror on my face, and I explained, "WE'VE LOST A SOCK! And Leta is wearing CUT-OFF DENIM PANTS, THAT ARE FRAYED AT THE END! MY MARRIAGE IS IN DANGER!"

Quickly we set out a plan of action: we would retrace our steps and look for the lost girly sock. Our chances of finding it were pretty good since the walk wasn't longer than a half mile. Chuck finally engaged in butt-sniffing and calmed down so that we could begin our walk home, and I kept shaking my head thinking, "Half-sockless, half-sockless, HALF-SOCKLESS!"

Not thirty seconds into our walk back home we spotted the missing girly sock lying in the middle of the sidewalk. My friend snatched it up from the ground and handed it to me, and I immediately put it in my back pocket and took off Leta's other sock. I wasn't going to risk losing a sock again, and so I continued the walk home with a totally sockless baby. Who was wearing frayed pants. We must have looked homeless and world-weary, me the crack-whore mother, Leta the crack baby.

My marriage had been saved.

A block before we got back to the house I got stung by a bee on my left hand. I was a little stunned, having just been through a half-sockless episode, and I swatted the bee away and pulled the stinger out of my thumb. THANK GOD I was the one who got stung because my friend was so allergic to bees that if she had been stung her lungs would have closed up and she might have died. If Leta had been stung, well, did Leta really need another reason to scream?

I wasn't normally allergic to bees, but my left hand swelled to the size of a grapefruit. It was so swollen that I couldn't even wear my wedding ring. So swollen that I looked like a crack-whore mother who got beat up real good in an alley behind the tattoo shop because I stole someone's needle. All while my sockless baby dangled like a large tumor from my chest.

Dear Leta,

Today you turn eight months old. We have several things to talk about, but the first and most important thing that we need to discuss are the two teeth that have taken residence in your mouth and in our house. Why did you have to go and grow those two teeth? Were they really necessary?

Perhaps the worst thing about your teeth is that they decided to sprout at the same time, which made your usual grouchy and cranky self a notch more grouchy and cranky, which in turn shook the foundation of the house and crumbled the brick exterior. I thought you were grouchy and cranky, but I had no idea what two teeth could do to a human being, and the world will never be the same. There is no wrath on earth as vengeful as the wrath of a teething baby, and I challenge anyone to stick their hand anywhere near your mouth without pulling it back missing a finger or two or five.

It's not like you really need teeth. You could sustain your life on milk and applesauce for years, and you can chew cereal with those two teeth just fine. Why grow more teeth when all that does is create more things to clean? You already have armpits and earlobes and fingernails that have to be cleaned, why add anything else? Take my advice: keep it simple. You'll thank me later.

Over the past month you have learned how to sit up by yourself. It happened overnight, like BOOM, there you were sitting there hanging out without tilting or leaning over. You have no idea how much this has contributed to our quality of life, as I don't have to carry you around kicking and screaming all the time. You can just sit there and kick and scream. I now have two free hands to do with whatever I want, like putting clothes on your head or taking a toy just out of your reach. OOOH, you can get testy, and you usually reprimand me by saying, "NA NA NA NA NA!" Which means, "Woman, my love for you is conditional, now give me back that goddamn toy."

You're constantly reaching for things and grabbing the remote or telephone out of my hands. You inspect objects like a scientist, end over end, and then you try to put things into your mouth from every angle. First the top of the thing goes into your mouth, then the bottom, and then the sides. One new object can entertain you for almost a half hour, but if you've already seen something you cannot be bothered with it. You've already seen that bunny! You've already played with that rattle! And this Tupperware container? You saw it TWICE yesterday. You get this really frustrated look on your face that says, "GOD, PEOPLE! CAN'T YOU BE MORE ORIGINAL? How big is this world that you brought me into, and these are the toys that you bring me? OFF WITH YOUR HEAD!"

You're now eating three meals a day in addition to the bottles we feed you, Oh Royal One. You love oatmeal and pears and sweet potatoes and apples and cereal, and last week we fed you pulled pork. You'll eat just about anything we feed you, and when we put food into our mouths we had better be prepared to share that food with you as you accost us with an open mouth, like a hungry baby bird. Your system is handling the new food well as you poop about forty times a day. One of the great mysteries of the Universe has to be how the hell I gave birth to such a regular baby.

Weekly physical therapy is going really well, meaning that you squawk less and less each week we put you through your exercises. You still refuse to put any weight on your legs, but the therapist thinks this may just be a characteristic of your personality rather than something neurological. When we distract you while we put you into certain weight-bearing positions you are fine, and then you realize, WAIT, we have distracted you and put you into a weight-bearing position and

WHO GAVE US PERMISSION TO DO THAT! SQUAWK! I'm working with you every day to get those chubby legs of yours to assume more responsibility, but this is a hard slog as you are so very stubborn. I can't blame you though; Jon Armstrong is your father.

Recently you spent two days with Grandmommy while your father and I "reconnected." I promise you will understand what that means when you have your own kids. When we walked into her house to pick you up you were sitting in the middle of her floor surrounded by cousins and toys, and both your father and I felt a rush of electricity shake us in our bones. We were so excited to see you, our little Scooter sitting there smiling, waving your arms and wiggling your hands. We never knew we could miss something so much.

We picked you up and hugged you, and then I handed you to your father so that I could go to the bathroom really quickly, and Leta, for the first time you cried as I turned to walk away. My mother assured me that you hadn't cried all weekend, but there you were, looking after me as I stepped closer to the bathroom, and gigantic tears fell from your eyes. I couldn't help myself, so I turned back around and scooped you out of your father's arms and took you to the bathroom with me. And there we were in Granny's bathroom, me on the toilet, you on my lap, smiling and peeing and being very much in love.

Love, Mama

CHAPTER SEVENTEEN

My Arms Spread Completely Wide

*C*huck had been in our lives for a little over two and a half years, and he'd always been a playful dog. Whenever we were on a walk people stopped to ask how old the puppy was because he looked like a puppy and would cuddle with anyone. We feared we might have over-socialized him as a puppy because he would play with any dog and then go over and say hello to the dog's owner as a courtesy and to see if there were treats to be had. PLEASE, SOMEONE, ANYONE, GIVE HIM TREATS.

Chuck and I had been reconnecting since I'd been home from the mental hospital, and he was living proof that dogs could read and respond to silent human emotion, although a lot of my emotion pre-hospital was of the non-silent, shrieking variety. As my postpartum depression got worse I would see less and less of Chuck throughout the day, and he never slept with us in bed, scared that I would throw him off of it one more time for making that annoying ball-licking noise. That has to be one of the world's worst noises, the slap-lapping of an empty nutsack by a dry dog tongue. My drugs may have been working but I still would have thrown him off the bed for that transgression, it was just THAT BAD.

Now that I was better—and let me just take a moment here to address just how much better I felt, I felt THIS much better, THIS being my arms spread completely wide, wide enough that I could hug every woman in the world who was suffering postpartum depression and let them know that things could get better—Chuck was at my side all day long, following me once again into every room, hinting that he wanted to go on another walk. We took naps on the couch together when Leta napped, his head usually pressed up against my feet. At night he roamed the kitchen with us as we made dinner, unafraid that I might throw a utensil or piece of burning food in his or Jon's direction.

I don't know if my depression sped up his aging process, but Chuck had become a crusty old man at the dog park and had taken to barking at more than his usual two things: 1) the neighbor, a taxidermist who came home smelling like fresh death every night, and 2) moving trash cans, specifically the ones we dragged from the backyard to the curb every Tuesday morning. I understood why he barked at the neighbor; the man killed and stuffed dead animals, animals closely related to Chuck in the evolutionary chart. In fact, I was surprised Chuck hadn't rounded up a group of neighborhood dogs to corner the man and take him out.

The moving trash-can thing was something I sort of trained him to do in a moment of complete stupidity. I thought it would be a fun game to play, having him chase me as I rolled the trash can to the curb. But he took it from chasing to nipping at my ankles to grabbing my pants leg to FULL ON BARKING AT ME. I couldn't even get near those cans without a glimmer of mischief sparkling in his eye, which had become problematic considering that I usually brought the cans back in from the curb while I was carrying Leta. It must have looked insane, that Armstrong woman with the sockless baby in one arm, her other arm pulling the trash can up the driveway, and that crazy dog running around her, biting her ankles and barking at her, all while she screamed CUT IT OUT, DOG. I MEAN IT. STOP. NOW. REALLY. STOP. STOP. WHAT DID I JUST SAY? STOP.

While Chuck got along really well with Leta—she loved to eat his tail and pat him on the back while she drank her bottle—he became jealous when we took her places and left him at home. We used to take him with us everywhere we went because that's what dumb, middle-class, childless people do when they have animals: they treat them like kids. How could we leave him at home, alone, for more than thirty minutes? He might get lonely! And need us! Why didn't our friends understand that when we came over for dinner parties WE HAD TO BRING THE DOG WITH US! He was a part of the family! Why didn't anyone shoot us in the head at close range?

Chuck was still very much a part of the family, but his role was now more that of a dog than that of a Prince who was heir to the family for-tune. When I ran errands with Leta I no longer stuck him in the back of the truck because we didn't have time to stop at the dog park, and that was just too much to handle: a cranky kid and a cranked-out dog. I'd usually pat him on the head and say, "You have to stay here and watch the house," because then I was giving him a job and don't dogs thrive on having a role in life? Isn't that what the dog books say, that dogs need jobs, that jobs make dogs happy? Well, Chuck never read that book, and when I left the house without him he thought I was saying, "I don't love you, and I have never loved you." Once I walked out the door and turned the lock he proceeded to find a way to take revenge, usually in the form of taking things out of the bathroom trash can, chewing them to pieces, and spreading them out on the bathroom floor.

Things that go into the bathroom trash can are by nature awful things containing awful fluids and awful waxes, so having them regurgitated and strewn about the floor was by nature unpleasant and punishable by death. But we loved Chuck, and the most harm we ever did to him was to bring him into the bathroom to the scene of the crime and shout NO! NO! NO! several times while hitting the toilet paper and tissue and half-chewed tampons. It was something our trainer in Los Angeles taught us to do, claiming that when we hit whatever the dog had chewed or destroyed we were creating a team with the dog against the object. The trainer assured us that it was much more painful for us than it was for the dog.

I once took an afternoon jaunt to the grocery store without Chuck in tow because hey! Dog owners! Dogs don't need to go to the grocery store! It's REVOLUTIONARY THINKING! I hadn't yet taken him on a walk that day for reasons I don't remember, so he was particularly pissed at me when I turned around to leave and said, "I've never loved you." Later that night, while Jon and I were eating dinner, Chuck brought us his victim clutched in his salivating jaws, Leta's green stuffed giraffe now missing both pink horns and a significant amount of stuffing. It was as if he felt so guilty about the crime that he brought it to us, his head hung low, his tail between his back legs.

Things were getting personal.

I knew that this was a bad case of separation anxiety and that we could improve the situation if we exercised Chuck more. But if given the choice between fetching an object or death from prolonged exposure to nuclear radiation, Chuck would have preferred the latter each and every time. He just wasn't born a fetcher, and that made exercising his bony ass somewhat tricky.

I tried to take him on at least one long walk a day, but when Leta insisted on being a big fat crybaby we stayed inside so that the neighbors didn't shoot me as I walked by. When Chuck didn't go on walks he got a raging case of cabin fever and then started to pace, and the endless clicking of his paws on the hardwood floors made me want to cut off his Frito-smelling feet and give Leta a few new toys to play with.

So we devised a game to exercise Chuck where Jon and I would stand at opposite ends of a field and shake bottles of pills. He'd hear the rattling of the pills and run between us to receive a treat. It was bribery, yes, and it worked.

One night the clicking of the paws was unbearable, and at about 9 PM we put on our coats, grabbed a couple of bottles of pills, and headed out into the front yard. Jon walked up the street and I rounded the house into the backyard, and we bribed Chuck to run between us about four times. The moon was out and shone bright through the haze of the valley's frost, and I looked down and noticed I was shaking a bottle of laxatives.

When we got back inside I checked Jon's bottle and smiled wickedly when I realized he'd been shaking a bottle of antipsychotics. Funny, he grabbed that one when he'd had the choice of four antidepressants, three antianxieties, two antiseizures, seven bottles of sleep aids, and one big container of stool softener.

One Saturday night we met my family for dinner at Chili's in Sandy, Utah, one of the more conservative patches of the Salt Lake Valley. I think it's pretty funny that I just wrote that, "more conservative patches of the Salt Lake Valley," as if people in one part of this place would give a better blow job to the Republican party than people who live a few blocks over. We had dressed Leta in her T-shirt that read, MOMMY WANTS A NEW PRESIDENT, risking a drive-by shooting if not a public hanging, and my mother said she had already seen that shirt, so she wasn't too shocked by it. That of course took away all the fun I had planned for the evening as nothing was more fun than shocking my mother. Yes, I was still that juvenile. Trust me, if your mom were the Avon World Sales Leader you would love to shock her, too.

I'm not usually a fan of chain restaurants, but I should probably come clean and confess the small place I have in my heart for Chili's: there is just something about their chips and salsa and willingness to bring two Diet Cokes at one time that make me forgive the aching heartburn that follows their meals. We were going to be arriving a little bit early to the dinner and Jon suggested we stop by a nearby bookstore to pass some time. I asked him why, and he said that he didn't want to get there too early so that we would have to sit there waiting for everybody while eating chips and salsa. AND WHAT WOULD BE WRONG WITH THAT? I couldn't follow his flawed logic and ordered him to drive straight there.

It was Leta's first family meal at a public restaurant where she would be sitting in a high chair all by herself. Before, we would hold her in our laps and eat merrily as she was too young to reach out and grab things. I remember having lunch with a friend and her two sons, ages three and one, when Leta was just three months old. Leta dozed in the car seat for the entire lunch while my friend's sons talked and GRABBED things and moved their bodies about in wholly acrobatic ways. I remember feeling horrified, that one day my baby would be big enough to shoot her arm across a table and grab something potentially spillable or just plain NOT HERS.

Of course, time passes and nightmares do come true.

Leta spent the entire evening grabbing her cousin Noah's things: his chips, his crayons, his sippy cup. My sister's twins, two of the most violent toddlers on earth, sat reverently in their high chairs staring in wonder as Leta pounded the table with her fists and grabbed everything within her wingspan. (The only reason I knew it was Noah and not Joshua was because she didn't dress them alike—very uncommon—and she identified them both when they arrived. Plus, the previous week I had gone to my sister's house, and when I pulled into her driveway I saw Noah climbing the mailbox in nothing but an undersized T-shirt—no pants and no underwear—and realized that he is the one who has the most self-inflicted bruises.)

Noah would occasionally turn to his mother and say very quietly, "She's taking my chips." Or, "She took my cup." I was watching her like a hawk, but she timed her illegal grabs right as I turned to take a chip and dip it into salsa. I had to clear a two-foot area around her high chair so that she wouldn't knock the table over with her banging, and that's when the public squawking started. Loud, piercing, bird squawks in between holding her breath and making her face turn red—I swear to God she was doing this, THROWING A PUBLIC TANTRUM. THIS WASN'T SUPPOSED TO HAPPEN FOR ANOTHER YEAR! I wanted my money back.

When you're childless and young and hopeful, you have this idea of what your children are going to be like, and you make mental notes when you see other kids in public. You say to yourself, "My kid will be cute like that," or "My kid won't ever throw a tantrum in public like that little demon." I had always envisioned a sweet little princess who looked just like me sitting quietly in a high chair, her pressed velvet petticoat creased perfectly as she sat and waited to be handed things in a timely manner. And then you grow up and have kids and realize that YOU HAVE NO SAY, and the only clean thing she can wear is that oversized red shirt that she will smear pears on before you leave the house, and that demon you once witnessed looks more and more human in hindsight.

One morning in late October it started to snow heavily, and as I was lurching in slow motion toward the window saying, *"OH MY GOD!"* the power went out. The lights turned off, the heat shut off, and worst of all, the television stopped working.

I immediately called my friend on the old phone in the basement to see if her power was out, too, and we joked and not joked about how important the television really was to us, and how in situations like that its importance was really driven home, and I realized that if it came down to the world not having television or me cutting off one of my feet I would totally give the world my foot. I love you, world, THAT MUCH.

I always had a television on in the house as background noise. It was crucial to my sanity to hear human voices during the day, even if those voices weren't talking to me and were badly acted as in the case of *Days of Our Lives.* That morning when the power went out I felt like someone had punched me in the gut, kidnapped all my friends, and then left me in a cold house with a baby who couldn't be entertained by any one thing longer than three minutes. And seriously, I was *this close* to running out of new things in the house to show her, *this close* to being me thinking twice that morning about getting out the 409 bottle and saying, "Here, Leta. This thing sprays!"

I had to gather my wits about me and come up with a quick plan: where could we go? We needed to go somewhere in the truck to stay warm and to kill some television-less time, but I couldn't think of anything we needed. We'd gone to the grocery store the day before (and the day before that, and the day before that), and all my prescriptions were filled, and I couldn't show my face at Old Navy ONE MORE TIME or they would think I was stalking them, WHICH I WAS.

And then I remembered! I needed moisturizer! And moisturizer required a car ride to procure! Off we went to an indoor mall far enough away that it hadn't been affected by the power outage, where there were horrible stores and horrible window displays full of Things You Don't Need including black plastic miniskirts and soaps in the shape of Joseph Smith's head. Were people really buying those plastic miniskirts? Because Hot Topic had at least two full racks of them, which meant they were stocking up for the Thanksgiving Plastic Miniskirt Rush, or no one was buying them, and the last time I checked the Mormons weren't wearing black plastic anything in public. And I'm sorry, but I'd have a hard time washing my crotch with a soap that was molded to look like a polygamous religious prophet.

I'd neglected to change out of my pajamas, and I was scurrying through the indoor mall with Leta on my hip, my pajama bottoms hanging sadly over the back of my running shoes. Certainly grounds for divorce. We raced to the only department store in the mall, the only place with those cosmetic counters manned by women whose faces look like they've had makeup tattooed on their eyes by a blind surgeon. We found the correct counter and I asked for my brand of moisturizer, and then the tattooed makeup lady, obviously surprised that someone so unkempt and still dressed in her pajamas would even know the importance of using moisturizer—so very, very, important, I had watched enough Bravo to know this—she said to me, "If you wait until Wednesday to buy this bottle of moisturizer you'll get a free gift."

FREE and GIFT in the same sentence? SIGN ME UP!

Turned out that the snowstorm would be sticking around for three more days, three days that I wouldn't be able to go on a walk and entertain the baby with the myriad of nontoxic outdoor things she hadn't yet seen. So I was going to need an excuse to get back into the warm car on Wednesday anyway. Was I a thinker, or what? So we drove all the way to the indoor mall for no reason, and I wasted gas and precious environmental resources, but that Wednesday I wouldn't have to come up with a plan, AND I'd get a FREE bag with extra eyeliner that I'd never wear!

That's called Professional Motherhood.

Utah celebrated Halloween on October 30 instead of the thirty-first because the actual holiday happened to fall on a Sunday that year. It's against the commandments to trick-or-treat on Sunday, as that would violate the commandment that says, "Thou shalt not celebrate the demonic holiday of Halloween on the Sabbath. But on any other day it's okay."

One precocious eight-year-old girl who was dressed as a large turtle came to our door and said, "Trick-or-treat. Happy Halloween TO-MORROW." And then she rolled her eyes as if she was being forced against her will to conform with all these morons. God made it snow all day on the thirty-first to punish anyone who didn't trick-or-treat the night before. He so wasn't kidding.

Our Halloween weekend started off with a bang at Jon's work Halloween party where we were witness to the part of Utah's population that refuses to practice birth control. There were more than three or four families there with eight or more children. That's the number that comes after seven, which is really six more than is allowed in some parts of the world. One family dressed their nine children as barn animals. I didn't know there were that many barn animals in the world, BUT THERE ARE. I sat for most of the party in Jon's cubicle with the little Leta Frog and let her play with the millions of things on his desk that she hadn't yet seen. She was entertained for a whole twelve minutes.

That night we attended a Halloween party at our friend Roger's house. Jon dressed as Drunkenstein, and I just went as Someone Who Wanted to Get Really Drunk. We stuck with gin all night, and I didn't make a huge fool of myself WHICH IS SAYING A LOT. I had a hard time not making a fool of myself at the parties at Roger's house, because he always had this table there with what seemed like thousands of liquor bottles, and I was allowed to pour my own drink and HOW CAN YOU POSSIBLY NOT GET INTO TROUBLE WITH THAT AROUND? I know that most normal people went to college parties where there were liquor tables, but I went to college in God's lap. Parties with liquor tables were a relatively new thing in my life, so in Liquor Years I was really only about twelve years old.

I was also trying to figure out who I was again, at least that was Jon's theory as to why I partied so hard when given a chance to party. Any time we had a chance to leave the baby at home and spend a few hours alone with people who spoke Adult I went a little nuts. Okay, a lot nuts.

On the Friday night following Halloween Jon put on his mod parka he got from a friend in 1985 when he was on a Mormon mission in Manchester, England, and I dressed up as lead singer Karen O of the Yeah Yeah Yeahs. My costume didn't involve much except black clothing, a lot of product in my hair, and really dark eyeliner. And I snarled a lot.

We went to an adult dress-up party, and I can't believe I just admitted that. It was a party, for adults, and we all dressed up like rock stars. I'm pretty sure that the whole thing was an excuse for the people throwing the party to send their three kids away for the evening, and for the rest of us to get away from our kids for the evening, with a pinch of trying to hold on to our fading coolness thrown in. The best part about the adult dress-up party, of course: the Free Tequila. If there were ever a badge of my cool days it would be how I could hold my tequila. And after that night there was no doubt that I STILL HAD IT.

No one could figure out my costume, of course, because everyone there stopped watching MTV before it was even invented, and if you're one of those few people who remember the days when MTV played videos then you're surely checking your hairline on a daily basis. We were all standing around the snack table when someone asked me to sing a song by the punk band, to demonstrate exactly who I was, and I shook my head no. "I'd rather not publicly embarrass my husband like that."

But Jon shrugged and told me to go for it, considering all the other times I had embarrassed him publicly, why stop now? So I put down the half-eaten cracker I had in my mouth, shook all my hair into the front of my face and shouted, "THEY DON'T LOVE YOU LIKE I LOVE YOU, MA-A-A-A-APS WAIT, THEY DON'T LOVE YOU

LIKE I LOVE YOU." And when I opened my eyes no one was saying anything or making any noise so I said, "Who knew maps could love you like that in the first place?" And then the room cleared. Public Embarrassment Number 2,124: ACCOMPLISHED.

Then we all went into the living room and played this music game where we split up into groups and had to name the song or name the artist or finish the next line in the song. Yes, it was a game. We were playing a game at a party. AND WE WEREN'T EVEN AT CHURCH. I should take a moment here to brag and let you know that I knew the answers to the ones about R.E.M., Electronic, Simon & Garfunkel, and The Carpenters. I even made up a line to a Carly Simon song and got away with it. I was on fire, I was smoking, I was DANGEROUS, and then they broke out all the music before 1975 and I had no idea what anyone was talking about. Even the woman who was wearing tapered, pleated jeans knew more than I did. Can someone please take a marker and write SHAM OF A HUMAN BEING on my forehead.

The best part of the night was when I went into their laundry room to say hi to their six-month-old terrier mix puppy, Jenny, who attacked me when I opened the door and proceeded to lick off my lipstick and all of my eyeliner. She was the happiest, most loving puppy in the entire world and since I'd had a portion of tequila normally seen only in my 2001 days, I got on the floor and had a huge puppy cuddle fest with that animal. It was purely platonic love, because I *was* married, and I was committed to a dog at home, and the Constitution prevents marriage between anything but a man and a woman and Jenny was not only not a human but she was also FEMALE.

I AM WHAT IS WRONG WITH THIS COUNTRY.

By the end of the night I had the dog in my lap and I was drunkenly singing, "THEY DONT LOVE YOU LIKE I LOVE YOU, MA-A-A-A-ATH, WAIT." And Jon was sitting next to me, his hand stroking the back of my head, and he leaned over and said, "I love going places with you." And if that was what being an adult meant, then kids, you've got so much to look forward to.

When Jon and I lived in Los Angeles we used to walk down to Damiano's Pizza on Fairfax every Friday night. It was just a couple of blocks from our apartment, and we always packed a flask of bourbon to see us on our journey. We'd order the pizza and then wait outside on the bench next to the storefront sneaking sips of bourbon and making friends with the local homeless people and members of the Russian Mafia.

One night we met an old Russian man named Abee, and oh the stories he had to tell! He was the type of man who wore a frown and tried to make you believe that being alive was the worst thing in the world, but you knew deep down that he loved people and that he'd take a bullet for you in a war.

Jon and I really warmed up to Abee, and we saw him several times on our drunken Damiano journeys. We'd see him and scream, "Abee!" and he'd scoff because that's what his role was, to scoff and be angry, but then we'd catch a small smile creep across his face. One Friday night Jon and I were talking to Abee and being terribly giddy and probably obnoxious in our drunkenness, and when Jon went inside to grab our slices I turned to Abee and said, "Man, *he's* crazy," referring to Jon and trying to get Abee on my side.

Abee immediately shook his head, scoffed again, and muttered in his Russian accent, "You make him that way."

And now, now whenever I nag Jon about something, something stupid because there's no need for nagging, he'll turn to me and say, in a fake Russian accent, "You make me this way!"

That shared history and his willingness to revisit it is one of the many reasons I cannot thank him enough for sticking with me, for not leaving when he would have been justified in leaving.

Jon and I used to go to the gym together in the morning before the baby was born. We used to do *a lot* of things before the baby was born, and going to the gym and staying awake past 10 PM were forced to the bottom on our list of priorities. I started to work out in the basement during Leta's first nap, by myself with a big bottle of water and a computer full of MP3s. We didn't have any exercise equipment, just a set of seven steep stairs that I'd go up and down five hundred times. And that last sentence just proves to you how insane the author really is.

I was always listening to music that Jon and I discovered together in LA, and so consequently, I was always reminded of my time in California when I ran the stairs in the basement: the crazy hours I used to work, the forty-five-minute commute to the office, the months that I dated Jason, Paul, August, Scott, Eric, Mark, and a few others whose memories were a little fuzzy, and thank God for fuzziness.

One morning in the middle of a workout while the baby slept upstairs, a Liz Phair song came on, and there was a line in that song that brought back the strongest memory of LA that I had, that of reconnecting with Jon and knowing that my life was going to change. It went: "But I can't imagine it in better terms/Than naked, half-awake, about to shave and go to work/I won't decorate my love."

In him I'd found the person whom I knew I would never get tired of, even in the most monotonous of times, even in the routine of being together every single day. I never thought I would find that.

I never thought I'd find the man who'd love to read my daughter her bedtime story, and one night after her bath as they sat cuddled together in her room reading Dr. Seuss books, I prepared a pan of Jon's favorite buffalo wings to put in the oven. I counted out six for me and six for him, and then I had a premonition and put one extra on the pan. Normally I would have just prepared the whole bag of fifty wings, but isn't there some saying about moderation in all things? Yeah, that's a dumb saying, but I wanted to be able to eat wings every night that week so I had to show some restraint.

Once they were out of the oven and cool enough to eat I ate my six and he ate his six in less than thirty seconds. And there sat that extra one I had put into the mix, and it sat there begging to be eaten. And Jon looked at me, and I looked at him, and he looked at me, and I looked at him, and this would have continued for infinity, but Jon finally asked, "How hungry are *you*?"

And I knew he needed that extra wing. That's why I had plucked it from the bag and placed it on the pan, because I knew that he was going to need that one extra morsel of Heaven. And I know that sometimes I am the most crass and awful person alive, but I love my husband. And I gave him that extra wing. It was my little way of saying, hey, I notice you didn't leave. Thank you.

Dear Leta,

Today you turn nine months old. This means that you have been outside of my womb for as long as you were inside it. At first it seemed you didn't like it on this side that much, but in the last month you have turned into one of the most giggly, tender, and joyous creatures that ever lived, at least when you're not screeching or trying to dig my eyes out of their sockets. That hurt.

When you were just weeks old and the transition in our lives was going a little haywire, people used to say to me, wait until she's three months old, or wait until she's six months old. Then, they said, things would be a lot better. Well, I waited and waited, and after the three- and six-month marks I was getting a little worried because you still seemed a little upset that I had taken away your placenta. But here at nine months, oh dear little Leta, we have hit that magical time when things are okay. This month I finally remembered why I wanted to procreate in the first place because you are just so cute that the frightening thought of one day trying to have another baby POPPED INTO MY HEAD, OH MY GOD. Someone please pinch me or throw water in my face and rid me of that nonsense.

In the last month we have met Leta The Person. You are no longer this little blob of a thing that I take care of and wipe up, but this flailing, wiggly little personality that likes certain things and really, really doesn't like other things. You love pears. You do not like peaches and will fling them at me if I try to feed them to you. You like applesauce. You do not like vanilla custard and you make this horrible gagging noise as it sits in your mouth and tries to make an innocent descent into your throat. You love to be tickled under your neck and around your thighs. You do not like it when I try to eat your nose and you'll look at me like, "Mom, that is so not cool. Get a grip."

In the last week you have discovered that if you throw yourself backward while sitting on my lap that the whole world turns UPSIDE DOWN! You LOVE to throw yourself backward and gurgle as you do it, and then you wait there for me to tickle you on your neck, and it is just the funniest thing in the whole world to you. If I'm late to tickle you on the neck you make this jerking motion with your body that seems to say, "Hey. Hey. You're supposed to tickle me on the neck now. Why are you veering from the routine?!"

We're still going to physical therapy to try to get you to put weight on your legs, but I think we're butting heads with the most stubborn part of your personality. You are not yet mobile; you aren't crawling or scooting or rolling across the floor. You're just very content to sit there surrounded by toys, and when you see other kids walking or crawling you stare at them like, "Why are they wasting such precious energy? Energy that could be used to rip apart a toy or scream for attention? Do they not know that EVERYTHING can be delivered right to them? That's what this whole baby thing is about." Right now I'm confident that you're going to be fine developmentally, that you'll eventually want something so badly that you'll move your body in its direction somehow. But I have to admit that having you immobile is somewhat convenient. I can turn my back and not worry that you'll be halfway across the room about to put your tongue into a light socket.

We finally have a solid routine during the day, one that can be timed by the clock, and you seem to like it just as much as I do. Within minutes of your naptime you show me signs of fatigue and make it solidly clear that you want nothing more than to curl up in your crib. The biggest sign that you are tired *is the rapid sucking of your thumb. Yes, the nightmare that people warned me about CAME TRUE: You are a thumb sucker! (That should be read as if God were yelling it down from the sky.) You suck your thumb, and surprisingly, THE WORLD STILL TURNS. The best part about your thumb sucking is, well, okay there are two best parts about your thumb sucking:*

1. *It takes you about three or four times to get your thumb into your mouth right. You'll bring it to your mouth, and then pull it away, and then bring it close again, and then pull away, like, "No, no, no, that's just not right!" The rest of your fingers caress your nose as you do this, and then finally, when you get your thumb into your mouth just right, your whole body relaxes like you've just taken a huge hit off a bong.*

2. *You suck your thumb rather loudly when you sleep. So loudly that we can hear it through the monitor, and your father is constantly telling me to turn that damn thing down. I like to hear it, because it lets me know that you are asleep and happy and snuggly with your friend, the thumb. But it is kind of an annoying noise, slurp slurp slurp, and I smile inside thinking about how horrified you would be if I recorded that sound and played it for your friends at your sixteenth birthday party. That is going to be so awesome.*

Today is a bit of a sad day for your father and me as the person we wanted to win the Presidency was defeated. It's sad mostly because we've brought you into a country that is heavily divided, and we're worried that things aren't going to get much better in your lifetime. We're leaving your generation a huge mess to deal with, but I want you to know now, here when your judgment isn't clouded by the crap that you'll hear on TV, here when your heart is pure, I want you to know that your father and I want to teach you love and compassion. We want to teach you that there are always several sides to every story. We want to teach you about all religions and let you choose for yourself what you want to believe. We want to teach you that there is power in knowledge, but that there is even more power in reaching out and loving other people, that life is about relationships and friends and giving everything you've got.

I love you, Leta. I love that you hug me tightly before I put you down for naps. I love it when you growl like a bear because you know that it makes me laugh. I love how you like to turn the pages in books. I love it that you cry when I leave and then brighten up like a sun-flooded room when I come back. I will always come back to you.

Love, Mama

CHAPTER EIGHTEEN

I Never Thought I Would
Become This Woman

A few days after Leta turned nine months old we shared a huge day full of doctor's appointments and cheddar cheese Goldfish. I had scheduled her physical therapy appointment after her first nap and her nine-month checkup after her second nap because I wanted her to be rested and in good spirits and an all-around lovely lady. You can do that as a parent, manipulate your children and ensure that they will be on their best behavior.

You, you who have children can now pick up your jaw after reading that last sentence, because it should be followed by a gigantic, witchlike cackle that goes something like, BWHA HA HA HA HA! YOU AND YOUR LITTLE DOG, TOO! For those of you who don't have children, the last sentence in the previous paragraph is the biggest bunch of bullshit I have ever spewed out of my mouth.

Leta was certainly going to be starting her period soon, because for several days she had been nothing but bipolar baby. I kept asking her to pick a mood and stick with it, because I felt like I was dodging bullets.

Thank God my meds were working because otherwise I would have been locked inside a closet on the phone with Jon, going, "SHE DOESNT EVEN LOOK LIKE ME," demanding that he come home from work so that I could get in the car, drive around the block with the windows down, and scream.

But the meds *were* working, so instead of crawling into the closet with the phone I was able to say, "Leta, all I did was take away my keys from you so that I could start the car. There is no need for your mouth to droop at the ends like that, and for that silent big breath before the storm of tears and screaming. Let's be civilized." That line of reasoning never worked, of course, and she cried and wailed, and couldn't understand why in the name of God I would be so audacious as to TAKE SOMETHING AWAY FROM HER. But babies have incredibly short attention spans, so once the wailing started I could hand her another object that had the potential to be taken away but was currently not in the state of being taken away. And did that ever shut her up.

The physical therapy session lasted forty-five minutes, which was a pretty long time for a nine-month-old baby whose normal daily routine was to sit, eat, burp, fart, and sleep. Leta's therapist worked her hard, and had her sitting in several weight-bearing positions, including one where Leta was sitting on a bench with her feet dangling off into a container of rice. This was supposed to help with sensory issues, and it was fascinating to watch as Leta leaned over and reached for the rice but then remembered, "My feet are down there and if I lean over I will have to put weight on them, and can someone tell me again why is that necessary?" That night as we were preparing Leta for bed I found rice in between her toes. And then the following morning I found rice in my bra. This is what happens when you have kids.

But we did get some good news; at her nine-month checkup we found out that Leta's head had grown significantly in the last month. The bad news was that the doctor must have measured her head wrong at the previous checkup (the checkup that had him so concerned that he ordered the MRI), that the little chart that illustrated the progress of her head circumference looked like it had been drawn by that guy I used to work with who was always so high on pot that HE FORGOT WHICH HAND HE WROTE WITH and used the wrong one.

Her head size was not even on the chart, it had grown so much. This meant that the piano in the dining room had to go because there was just too much mass in our area of the neighborhood, what with Leta's head in the room, that our house was in danger of turning into one big black hole and sucking the entire state into its abyss. Good-bye, Utah! Hello, one less red state!

A few days later she woke up at 5:30 AM making her usual noises that say, "hey, I'm awake now, come and get me this instant." This happened from time to time, and our usual response was to let her fall back asleep until 7 AM so that we could start our day on schedule. Usually she complied and fell back asleep, but that morning she was being really obstinate and her noises were more like, "NO, SERIOUSLY, COME AND GET ME NOW."

So Jon went to check on her to see if everything was okay, but he didn't have his glasses on or his contact lenses, which meant an elephant could have been sitting in Leta's crib and he wouldn't have seen it. He came back to bed and said, "All her limbs are in place, she'll go back to sleep." Seconds later her noises escalated to, "THAT'S IT, I'M PRESSING CHARGES."

So I climbed out of bed and went in to see what was going on, and what Jon didn't see was that Leta had turned ninety degrees from the direction we had put her to sleep in the night before. She was perpendicular, and her head was stuck up against the bumper, her feet kicking the bumper on the opposite side, her entire body out from under the covers. The eerie thing about the whole situation was that her blankets appeared as if they hadn't moved all night; they were perfectly straight, exactly as we had covered her the night before. It was as if some unknown force had entered her room in the middle of the night, picked her up, and placed her at the head of her crib in the wrong direction.

I yelled, "Jon! You've got to come see this," and Leta looked up at me like, "How did this happen?" And I was all, "Dude, you're the one who got yourself into this mess, explain it TO ME."

I could barely handle the thought. It meant she was on the verge of mobility. She was on the verge of being able to move from point A to point B, which meant that the purchase of plastic outlet covers was upon us. PLASTIC. OUTLET. COVERS. Who came up with that whole concept? Some baby somewhere was sticking his tongue into an outlet, and his parent had to go, "Dude, I've got an idea, and we are so going to be rich." And I was going to be putting money into that person's pocket. All because our baby just had to go ahead and be mobile.

And yet, maybe our baby would one day be mobile! Holy shit, *it just might happen.*

Two weeks later we were at a dinner party when one of the neighbors I had never met walked up to Leta and me and asked how old she was. When I told him she was almost ten months old he asked if she was walking all over the house yet. I answered, simply, "No."

He looked quite surprised and then continued, "Well, I guess she must be in that crazy crawling stage, huh?"

And when he said that, it felt like a dagger went through my heart. I explained, "Actually, she isn't crawling, either. She has some sensory problems and refuses to put any weight on her legs." And then I wanted to run out of that house, Leta pressed to my chest, and go hide with her under the covers in the bed.

It's not that I was ashamed of the fact that she wasn't crawling. It's just, people asked me all the time why she wasn't crawling yet, and I felt like I was doing something wrong. I felt like it was my fault, and while I knew that wasn't true, I kept wondering if there was something I should have been doing that I wasn't doing. We saw a physical therapist every week, and I worked with her every day on her exercises. Still, it hurt me to hear her scream when I forced her to move in ways she didn't like to move.

This was part of being a mother, I suppose: the constant nagging feeling of guilt and sorrow and joy and worry and unfettered elation, feelings that should not exist simultaneously but CONSTANTLY EXIST SIMULTANEOUSLY.

I had never been so alive, and yet, so on the verge of collapse.

A few weeks before Leta turned ten months old a neighbor came over on a Saturday morning so that Jon could walk her through a design software application. Jon is THAT person, the one you turn to for any and all technical questions and has helped members of my family and his family and neighbors and plumbers with questions about their computers. For all the time he has spent walking my father through The Microsoft Blue Screen of Death we should have wiggled our way back into my father's will, or at least have made it back onto the list of people he wants to attend his funeral.

Leta had taken a terrible first nap, and by terrible I mean not long enough to mask her inner raging beast. This happened a lot, and what I had to do was keep to our schedule and make sure she took her second nap at the precise time so that we could correct the balance of the universe, because if she took a bad second nap . . . do you remember that movie *The Day After*? Where the world has been obliterated?

Jon knew not to question me when I went into Project Prevention of Leta Fallout Disaster Mode, a finely tuned ballet where I distracted the living shit out of that kid and brought her delicately to the crescendo of her second nap where the violins and cellos trembled in unison and hummed her softly into a deep, soul-cleansing sleep that would leave her refreshed and bearable to be around. Sometimes the only way to do that was to leave the house, and since Jon was teaching our neighbor about the various ways you could crop the head off of someone's body in a photograph, I had to go on this adventure alone.

ALONE. (ECHO ECHO ECHO)

So I packed up the kid and headed to my P.O. Box because I couldn't think of anything else to do. We'd done all our grocery shopping and had been to Costco earlier in the week. (Just a note here: for those dead souls out there who refer to Costco as "The Costco," may a house fall out of the sky onto your head and your legs shrivel up underneath it.) My P.O. Box happened to be in an area surrounded by other shops including a Starbucks, and you know what they sell at Starbucks? SUGAR. So the mailbox seemed like a good idea. Sugar + mail + distracted kid = One Badass Mother.

And here's the point in the story where my ego begins to unravel.

The first mistake I made was to park the car in front of the building that housed my P.O. Box, because that building was all the way over to one side and not at all close to any of the other shops. But that didn't matter at the time. I was going to get actual mail, that I could hold in my hands, and it felt like Christmas. The rush was a little blinding. And because I didn't think we would be gone for a very long time I just held Leta on my hip. Because my brain was made of Skittles.

Inside the mailbox was a gift from a friend for Leta, a pair of shoes to help keep her socks on. One pair had frogs on the toes, and I opened the package right there and put the shoes on her feet immediately. Enter mistake number two, stage left. Leta screamed the entire time I manipulated her feet into the shoes as if I were severing her feet from her body. Not because it hurt, but because she didn't want to move her feet the way I needed her to move her feet and CURSE YOU, ARMSTRONG GENES.

We headed back to the car to drop off the packaging so that I wouldn't have to carry it around, and that's when I should have come back to my senses. Why didn't I just get back in the car and drive over to the Starbucks? BECAUSE THAT WOULD WASTE GAS AND JUST SCREAMS LAZINESS, RIGHT? But that's not why I didn't get back into the car. I didn't get back into the car because I calculated the amount of energy it would take to carry her over to the Starbucks versus the energy it would take to put her into her car seat again, strap her in, start the car, drive over, and GET HER BACK OUT, and my math told me that if I had to do and undo that car seat buckle one more damn time I might say horrible words in front of my innocent daughter. I did it for her.

So we began the walk, and it was a walk and a half, not unlike how Moses led his people through the desert, onward and onward, not unlike how the Mormon pioneers trekked across the plains. We walked and walked, or shall I say I walked and walked, and Leta bobbed up and down on my hip, and all of a sudden I remembered, SHIT! One of the neighborhood kids was having a birthday the following week and we didn't have a present for him yet. And the Old Heather flew down from the sky and sat on my shoulder and whispered, "That's okay, you've got the rest of the weekend to go and get something. Relax." But the new Heather, the Mother Heather, the daughter of the Avon World Sales Leader Heather who was coming into her birthright, this new Heather ROARED from the inside of my body and made my head spin around three times.

The Mother Heather reasoned, "WE ARE HERE. TOY STORE RIGHT THERE. PRESENT MUST BE BOUGHT NOW." And I couldn't stop myself. I COULDNT PROCRASTINATE. I had to get that birthday present right then because it MADE SENSE. OH GOD, what had I become? And as I walked into the toy store and found an age-appropriate, nonflammable present the Old Heather took her devil wings and forked tail and shook her head in disgust as she flew off my shoulder.

So with Leta on my right hip and a large present hanging in a bag from my left hand I walked over to the Starbucks. FINALLY. And the end was in sight, it really was, I could see the light, but that's when Leta started to squawk. Loudly. In public. And the motherly instinct kicked in once again and I reached for my keys and shoved them into her mouth and she couldn't have been more delighted. And so we were standing there in the middle of Starbucks, Leta with half of a Nissan remote-control door-opener hanging out of her mouth, the present now half-hanging out of the bag, and I couldn't reach my wallet in my back pocket. Why don't mothers come with four hands? TELL ME WHY.

So I sat Leta on the countertop to reach for my wallet, and at that moment she dropped the keys. And even though it was her fault that the keys were no longer in her mouth—IT WASN'T MY FAULT—she began to scream. And right then the present fell out of the bag. And I fumbled to get the wallet out of my pocket, and the moment I brought it in front of me Leta snatched it and grabbed the cash hanging out of the side and stuck it into her mouth.

Dirty, dingy, germ-infested money, in my baby's mouth. At least she was no longer screaming.

It was in that moment, that horrible, chaotic, sweat-on-my-upper-lip moment, that I looked with pleading eyes at the sixteen-year-old barista and said, "No, seriously, I never thought I would become *this* woman."

The weekend before Thanksgiving my sister's neighbor committed suicide. He was the father of four children, the oldest being eleven, the youngest being three, and his wife found him in their bedroom where he had hanged himself.

When my sister called to tell me about it I almost collapsed onto the floor. That could have been me. It could have been Leta who was left without a parent, Jon without a partner. If cameras had been following me around during those awful months of my postpartum depression you would have seen me throwing full gallon milk jugs at Jon's head. You would have watched as I slammed the front door so hard that it fell off of its hinges, or the countless number of times I called Jon at the office just so that I could hang up on him. Maybe you would have seen me through the window as I stood in front of the medicine cabinet in the kitchen trying to figure out whether or not I had the nerve to take an entire bottle of Risperdal.

I thought about suicide every day during those months. I thought about how I would do it; perhaps I would hang myself with the dog's leash, or maybe I'd grab every single pill we had in the cabinet and drown them with a couple shots of tequila. I wanted to do something, anything to stop the pain.

But I finally gave in and realized that I couldn't climb out of the hole by myself, and I had come to accept that I would continue to take medication for the rest of my life. I would never be off medication. I continued to see my therapist, not every week or even every month, but whenever I hit a road block and needed someone to help me talk my way through it. Sometimes I had bad days, sometimes bad weeks, but the medication enabled me to cope, to see a way out and over those times. I was not ashamed of any of this.

I knew so many people who were afraid that if they took medication or even agreed to see a therapist that they were in some way admitting failure or defeat. Or they had been told by their boyfriend or their mother or their best friend that they should buck up and get over it, and that asking for help was a sign of weakness. Well then, let me be weak. Let me be a failure. Because being over here on this side, where I could see and think clearly, where I was happy to greet my child in the morning, where I could logically maneuver my way over tiny obstacles that would have previously been the end of the world, over here being a failure was a hell of a lot more enjoyable than the constant misery of suffering alone.

All of this is to say that I was a success story. I was a victory for the mental health profession. And despite everything that it would say about me and who I was to have to ask for help, I did it. And here was this crazy woman in the Utah desert who admitted and accepted all of those horrible things about herself and in doing so found a better life.

That night as Jon and I got Leta ready for bed we went through the routine in silence as both of us rolled around thoughts of my sister's neighbor in our heads.

"You know, this lotion," I said to him as we rubbed a lavender-scented moisturizer into the folds of her chubby legs, "it reminds me of the hospital and the four days I spent there."

He looked up at me immediately. "I'm sorry," he said. "We can buy a different lotion if this is too painful for you."

"No," I said. "It's actually a great memory. You would come to visit me, and whenever you brought Leta she smelled exactly like this. I'd scoop her out of the stroller and press my nose against her forehead so that I would remember that smell after you took her home."

"You remember that?" he asked.

Yeah, I remembered that. I remembered how they came to see me every day. I remembered how neither of them gave up on me.

I didn't wash my hands after putting the lotion on Leta's body, and after we put her to bed and for the rest of the night I would sneak quick sniffs of my hands. I realized that this smell would always remind me of Life.

Afterword

October 2009

As I sit here typing this, five years after living through the early months of my first child's life, I am holding my second baby, another girl, and her smile is so wide that it barely fits in the room. I remember once thinking that the logistics of handling two children would be more complicated than quantum physics, and that I would never evolve to a place where I would even be willing to try for another child, would never want to risk living through postpartum depression ever again. And then my first child threw her first three-year-old tantrum, and the agony of postpartum depression seemed minimal in comparison.

Leta, my first daughter—you may know her as Her Screamness Who Screams A Lot Every Day With The Screaming—continued to have delays in her gross motor development throughout the first three years of her life. After a second MRI to determine that nothing was wrong with her spine, we enrolled her in a few Early Intervention programs that involved occupational and physical therapy to help her process sensory information in a less painful way. She didn't walk until she was almost two, didn't run until she was almost three, couldn't jump until she was almost four. And in the meantime the screaming never really stopped. There was never an official diagnosis, only that we had given birth to an incredibly stubborn child who seemed to delight in the agony of her parents.

Now at five and a half years old she is reading on a third-grade level and could easily argue a case in front of the Supreme Court. We have decided to keep her.

Leta apparently takes after her father's youngest sister, and many times I have heard Jon's mother say that if her last child had come first she wouldn't have had any more children. That was our thinking for at least three years; that our unit was complete and we'd be insane to combine our DNA yet again. But sometime during her fourth year when Leta's screams turned into articulate sentences, I realized just how far we'd come, just how much easier and better it was. And I remembered that so many people had said that this would happen. At that point I could see the trajectory clearly, and suddenly the possibility of trying again started popping up at the dinner table, during our morning routine, at lunch, and then in every other sentence.

"What you're telling me is you want another baby," said Jon one night as I rubbed my snotty, tear-stained face all over his T-shirt, a crying jag brought on by a commercial for Viagra. What? I see the connection very clearly.

Yes, I wanted another baby, but even more than that I wanted the chance to *enjoy* one, because my depression had robbed me of so many of the precious moments of Leta's early months. The anxiety over her endless screaming, over whether or not my breast milk supply was enough to sustain her, over what would happen if I turned my back for a single moment—it stole her infancy from me. And now that I was on the other side of it, now that I had the tools and knowledge of having lived through it, I wanted another chance.

Jon and I are fortunate to be so fertile that I can get pregnant just by lying next to him in bed fully clothed, and in the fall of 2007 we once again saw that second line on a pee stick. We immediately contacted my OB-GYN and asked her advice concerning pregnancy and medication. She suggested that I stay on my antidepressant, so I did, and those first few weeks were marvelously uneventful. In fact, I didn't experience any of the morning sickness that I'd had with Leta, and we eagerly began planning for the exciting changes in our lives.

At the beginning of the eleventh week of that pregnancy, just a few days before announcing it to friends and family, I started spotting and an unplanned ultrasound showed that the baby had died a few weeks earlier. I was given instructions to go home and let my body take care of things naturally. For a week I holed myself up in our bedroom, waiting for the inevitable, crying and grieving the loss of what could have been, the infant I would never know. And then it happened, I experienced a miscarriage like so many other women, an unspeakable pain, the details of which no one should ever have to live through.

I was scared after that experience to try for another pregnancy, mainly because I didn't know if I could survive that kind of grief should something go wrong again. But even if I had wanted to try right away, my body made other plans and took several months to get back to normal. A year later we made our first attempt at another baby, and that is when our beautiful Marlo Iris was conceived.

My pregnancy with Marlo was similar in so many ways to my pregnancy with Leta: the morning sickness, the aches and pains, the weight gain, the (ahem) hemorrhoids. But I remembered the advice of my doctors and remained on my antidepressant throughout. And then in my thirtieth week I read a transforming book about natural childbirth and decided to prepare myself to deliver our second child without any drugs or interventions. Those next ten weeks of my pregnancy were some of the most peaceful weeks of my entire life, and never before did I feel so in touch with who I was and what I wanted in life.

On June 14, 2009, Marlo's actual due date, I gave birth to the quietest, most gentle little girl after only three and a half hours of terrifyingly painful drug-free labor. The adrenaline rush from natural childbirth was not unlike snorting an entire eight-ball of cocaine, and for two days straight I remained awake, alert, and so in love with that baby. For two days she was attached to my chest and I did nothing but marvel at her every feature. That fascination with her has never changed, and neither Jon nor I have experienced any of the shock that we did when we brought Leta home. Breastfeeding was so much easier this time. In fact, it was an absolute joy, and both Jon and I could change a diaper with one hand while multi-tasking with the other. There was none of the crazy stress that was there when our lives shifted from childless couple to Family of Three.

However, on day three something happened. At first I thought it was the sleep deprivation catching up with me, so I ignored it. But by day five and six I couldn't pretend I was okay anymore. I started having panic attacks and such severe anxiety that my hands started to contort and clutch into twisted positions that I could not relieve. I couldn't fall asleep or stay asleep, and my mind started spiraling into dangerous places. I was so angry, so frustrated because there was no reason to feel this way. Intellectually I knew everything was okay, and *my god! I knew what I was doing!* I loved the baby and knew how to meet her needs!

There just wasn't a good explanation for my crippling anxiety, but there it was. And it was robbing me of the experience I was determined to have.

So we immediately called the doctor who treated me for the postpartum depression I had with Leta. He does not normally see patients who are not in the hospital, but by some lucky twist of the universe he thought I was someone else, someone whom he owed a favor, and agreed to see me as an outpatient. Two days later I was sitting there on a couch in his office facing him as he contorted his face in an effort to figure out just who the hell I was. And I was sweating, the anxiety crawling slowly up my body and paralyzing my neck. For several agonizing, silent minutes he scrolled through files on his computer until he found mine from five years ago. And as he glanced at me and then back at his computer, I involuntarily blurted out, "I wrote a book about my experience in the hospital." Maybe to let him know that I was serious? That here I was dumb enough to try and do this whole thing again? And he immediately whipped his head around and said, "You're THAT woman?"

Yes. Indeed. THAT woman. The woman who writes about poop and hemorrhoids and stitches in her vagina YES DEAR GOD THAT'S ME. Listen, my Republican, Mormon, gun-owning father read my book and he still loves me! That counts for something, right?

Turns out that his wife had heard about my book, and when she was describing it to him he knew immediately that I had to have been someone he treated because of the speed with which I healed. He treats postpartum depression very differently than most doctors, and his patients usually see results instantly. And that is exactly what happened with me in the hospital five years ago: I took a cocktail of meds and within two hours I felt like a different person.

So we did a lot of talking, and since he's been treating women for this very condition for over thirty years I did a lot of listening and learning. The odds were completely stacked against me, and he said that if I had been gearing up and treating the possibility of this with the right combination of medication in my third trimester I might have been able to avoid it. But since I didn't it was time to attack it now. So he made a minor tweak to my meds and asked me to come back and see him in two weeks, and I am not even kidding, I felt better that night. In fact, better does not do justice to what I was feeling. I felt *free.*

I've been on the new meds since that afternoon a few months ago, and I haven't had a panic attack once. I feel like a regular person who has an infant and can handle it, and during my pregnancy that was exactly what I was aiming for. Turns out I needed a little help, a tiny adjustment, but here I am and I am loving it. I love what it has done to my relationship with Leta, what it has helped me see and appreciate in Jon, and I love that I can barely stand to be away from that baby for a minute. I have been present for all her coos and giggles, for all the funny faces and exploding diapers, for all the quiet, glorious moments in the middle of the night when she wakes up and I feed her. I got my second chance.

Acknowledgments

I want to thank my agent, Betsy Lerner, who had no idea what kind of mess she was getting into when she sent me that letter four years ago. We have been through a war together, with gaping scars to prove it, and it speaks volumes about her character that she didn't abandon me on the side of the road. Her vision and encouragement are directly responsible for the fact that I survived the act of putting this book together. I owe her a beer.

Many thanks to my editor, Patrick Price, who has nothing in common with me and yet still laughs at my dick jokes. I feel like he looked directly into my heart and understood me immediately. I am forever indebted to the patience he showed in dealing with such a novice.

Thanks also go to Radiohead, Beck, Justin Vernon of Bon Iver, Neko Case, and Wilco, whose music cured some serious bouts of writer's block.

I want to thank my daughter's babysitter, Katey Kendall, for giving me the free time to find the mind that I had lost, and also for being the little sister I never had.

Thanks to my mother, Linda Hamilton-Oar, The Avon World Sales Leader, she who gave me the brains and the brawn to fight my way through anything. I remember in the hours after my daughter's birth finally understanding the look I had seen in my mother's eyes so often, and I thank her for forgiving me for being the reason behind it.

Thanks to my father, Michael Hamilton, for his ongoing support, especially for being willing to believe that what I went through was real.

Thanks to the readers of my website who sent me messages of hope during what were the darkest months of my life. Without them I would not be alive.

Finally, I want to thank the two most important people in my life: Jon Armstrong, my soul mate, he who did not leave me when he had every reason to do so. This book is a love letter to him.

And Leta, my beautiful daughter, the most stunning force of nature I've ever encountered, my muse. I want to thank her for letting me share this story so that others might not feel so alone.